myoActivation Explained

For people experiencing chronic
pain and myofascial dysfunction.

Dr Liesl Roome, MBChB, CCFP

◆ FriesenPress

One Printers Way
Altona, MB R0G 0B0
Canada

www.friesenpress.com

Author: Dr Gillian Lauder
Author: Barb Eddy

ISBN
978-1-03-832822-9 (Hardcover)
978-1-03-832821-2 (Paperback)
978-1-03-832823-6 (eBook)

1. MEDICAL, PAIN MEDICINE

Distributed to the trade by The Ingram Book Company

For people experiencing chronic pain and myofascial dysfunction

Dr. Liesl Roome

Table of Contents

Foreword

—by the originator of myoActivation,
Dr Greg Siren MD FCFP, Victoria, BC, August 22, 2024

This book is another step forward to expanding knowledge about myoActivation for patients and their supporters. Thanks to Liesl Roome, Barb Eddy, Gillian Lauder, and others who made the effort to bring this information together in printed form!

The myoActivation methodology evolved from techniques I learned in the late 1990s from a good physician friend when I was working in the US as an urgent care doctor. The techniques he taught me were based on Travell and Simons' *Myofascial Pain and Dysfunction*. I started using these techniques in practice and found that many of my patients living with chronic pain would get relief.

Over time, with careful examination and observation, using palpation as a guide, I noticed that the source of pain often was distant from the body location where the patient felt it. What evolved was a series of movement tests that helped identify impairments and allowed me to isolate the true source of pain. I also noticed the dramatic changes in patient's pain and dysfunction with the treatment of scars.

My interest in refining the assessment and treatment approach further accelerated in 2009 when I was the physician on board oil rigs relocating across the Atlantic Ocean. During these two-month cruises, I treated rig workers living in pain while still working twelve-hour shifts.

As I lived in close quarters with these workers, I noted the positive changes in mood, social interaction, and activity as their pain and dysfunction diminished with treatment. I was so impressed with the results I observed I decided to open a clinic and concentrate on developing this technique. As a result, the myoClinic launched in early 2010 in Victoria.

Since then, I've worked on evolving the methodology with the goal of teaching myoActivation to other clinicians so as many patients as possible can benefit from it. The vision is to treat people early in their pain journey to avoid escalation of their pain and dysfunction and perhaps also the eventual need for surgery or other invasive treatments.

None of this would have transpired without the encouragement and support of my wife, Judy Pryce. Judy was the muse for the early development of the methodology and the financial, legal, and editing master underpinning this work.

Since opening the clinic, some notable advancements have included:

- The use of pre- and post-treatment movement testing during a session. This allows patients to clearly sense changes resulting from treatment and identify any further areas for future treatment if needed.
- Incorporating findings from further study in the anatomy and physiology of fascia, the thin connective tissue that surrounds and supports every part of the body. Tight, thickened, or tethered fascia can restrict movement and cause many painful health conditions.
- Development of a formal training curriculum for clinicians, including four levels of skills training in increasing levels of complexity.
- Working with specialists in various areas to address "pain conundrums" that may persist in cases after their typical therapies have not been fully successful. For instance, we have worked with specialists in urology, physiatry, psychiatry, neurology, general surgery, and others.

- Establishing a non-profit entity, the Anatomic Medicine Foundation (www.anatomicmedicine.org), to allow for continuing development of the method.

So far we have been focusing our training efforts in British Columbia, and more clinicians have been offering this treatment option to patients.

But there is still so much more to be done! I believe that myoActivation is a low-risk and simple procedure that is effective for most patients, allowing them to live with less pain and dysfunction, without drugs. Future developments I would hope to see include:

- myoActivation as a basic skill of any healthcare professional delivering primary care who is licensed to use needles.
- Expansion of the procedure across Canada and other countries as well.
- Collaboration with various medical specialties to support their patients where pain symptoms may have myofascial origins.
- Development and delivery of education about myofascial pain solutions to patients and their communities.
- Promotion of scientific research relating to drug-free treatments of myofascial dysfunction.

Thanks to everyone working toward developing any of these ideals!

Author's Foreword

I learned the myoActivation methodology from Dr Siren starting in 2016. A doctor had covered my practice for a few weeks while I was away, and when I returned, patients demanded I learn to do the trigger point injections he was doing. This started my journey with myoActivation.

As I started implementing these treatments into my everyday practice and witnessing their effectiveness, I felt it was a field that really could make a substantial difference in patient's lives. We were amid a global crisis as far as opiate use was concerned, and there was not much to offer patients in chronic pain as an alternative. I started doing a few days a week at the myoClinic in Victoria and was doing myoActivation full-time in 2018. During the pandemic in 2020, Dr. Siren stepped back from clinical practice, and the myoClinic Brentwood Bay was started to continue the work. I have now completed over 34000 patient encounters in the last 6 years, and the consistency of results and patient outcomes still continue to impress and surprise me.

I have found daily, that patients want to know more about myoActivation, how it works, what fascia is, what to do after treatment etc. and felt that I needed to put it all together and have the information available as a resource. I think myoActivation is an option that the world needs and I hope this publication will help to explain it.

I want to thank everyone who contributed to the text: Dr G Siren, Dr Gillian Lauder, and NP Barb Eddy; as well as, Dr Kurt Dreschner, NP Carrie Murphy, Tanja Crowie, and Anel Visser for their insights.

Abbreviations

3P   physiotherapy (and massage), psychology, pharmacology

BASE   biomechanical assessment and symmetry evaluation

IMS   intramuscular stimulation

MFD   myofascial dysfunction

PRP   platelet-rich plasma

TiLT   timeline of lifetime trauma

Introduction

Key points

- This book is about myoActivation, a new therapy that can help with chronic pain. The book is designed to explain how myoActivation could help you with your pain.
- Each section will start with a simple list of the main points. It will highlight the key takeaways.
- There are sources at the end of the book for readers who want to learn more, both individuals suffering from chronic pain and doctors who want to learn how to give this treatment.
- myoActivation was created by Dr. Gregory Siren. He also created the Anatomic Medicine Foundation to keep improving the treatment.

myoActivation®, developed by Dr Gregory Siren, is a simple, low-cost, medication-free technique that can help with various chronic pain issues.

Dr. Siren trademarked myoActivation® (the small "m" and the capital "A" are intentional as this is a trademarked name) to preserve intellectual property and the unique standardized process of this treatment; he also started a non-profit foundation to refine the treatment, educate doctors and patients, and make it more accessible. To explore his not-for-profit, the Anatomic Medicine Foundation, visit its website: www.anatomicmedicine.org.

This book is designed to help patients living with pain, understand what myoActivation is and address expectations for myoActivation therapy. Wherever possible, evidence-based explanations will detail the effects of myoActivation on the different tissues.

It can be difficult for a person living with constant or severe chronic pain to retain large amounts of information, so this book is portioned into short sections that address key questions about myoActivation.

Since some readers may want answers to only a few questions and may not want to read it from beginning to end, key messages will be highlighted in the key points section at the start of each chapter. These sections use plain language to outline important content from a patient's perspective. There may also be some repetition of key points for those who only read a chapter or two.

While the main aim is to provide a helpful introduction for myoActivation patients, references will be included to be informative to those who would like more information, including medical professionals who may want to determine if myoActivation could help their patients.

With greater knowledge and understanding of the process, the hope is that patients can derive the maximum therapeutic benefit from myoActivation treatments.

Chapter 1: What is myoActivation?

"The best treatment I ever had; I already feel so much better."

—myoActivation patient who had severe lower back pain

Key points

- myoActivation uses movement tests and medical history to determine where pain originates.
- If the movement tests cannot be done, the clinician (a doctor or nurse) can assess you as you lie down.
- The place that hurts may not be the source of your pain. Because everything in the body is connected, the real problem might be somewhere else.
- The clinician will put a thin, sharp needle into the spot that's causing your pain. Putting in the needle is called "needling."
- The needle will be empty or have a little salt water in it.
- The spot that is causing your pain might be a scar, a tight muscle, or a tissue in the body called the "fascia."
- myoActivation includes movement tests, some needling, and then more tests to see if you need more treatment.

Understanding myoActivation and myofascial dysfunction

Myofascial dysfunction—when the muscles ("myo") and the connective tissues ("fascia") aren't functioning together as they should. This is a common yet often overlooked component of chronic pain. When you feel pain in a particular part of the body, the true source of pain may be located elsewhere. This may seem surprising, not only to the person living with pain but also to many healthcare practitioners. For example, a C-section scar (from childbirth surgery), which is located on the lower abdomen, can sometimes cause strain to the back muscles. In these cases, myoActivation can relieve low back pain and improve mobility by releasing the tension around the scar.

The process of myoActivation

myoActivation is a system that has its own unique assessment and treatment process.[1] [2,3] The technique uses a very fine hypodermic needle (thin needle designed to inject substances or withdraw fluids beneath the skin) to release tight muscles, fascia, and scars. The goal is to release the myofascial dysfunction that is the true source of pain.

Unlike conventional medical history-taking, the myoActivation assessment establishes a detailed history, known as the timeline of lifetime traumas (TiLT). TiLT includes a comprehensive account of previous injuries, surgeries, physical traumas, burns, broken bones, bad falls, tailbone injuries, illnesses, or anything that may have created scars on and within the body.

After the TiLT is completed, a myoActivation clinician (myoClinician) carries out a postural assessment. During this stage, the myoClinician asks the patient where they feel pressure under their feet to determine weight distribution, which gives insights into the body's centre of gravity. Next, the clinician proceeds with careful observation of the symmetry of the body, including the positioning of the feet and knees, orientation of the hips and shoulders, and establishing where the head is positioned relative to the neck and shoulders.

Biomechanical assessment and symmetry evaluation (BASE tests)

This observation is followed by specific movement tests called the biomechanical assessment and symmetry evaluation (BASE tests) to identify areas that need treatment. Some of the core movements are shown in Figure 1.

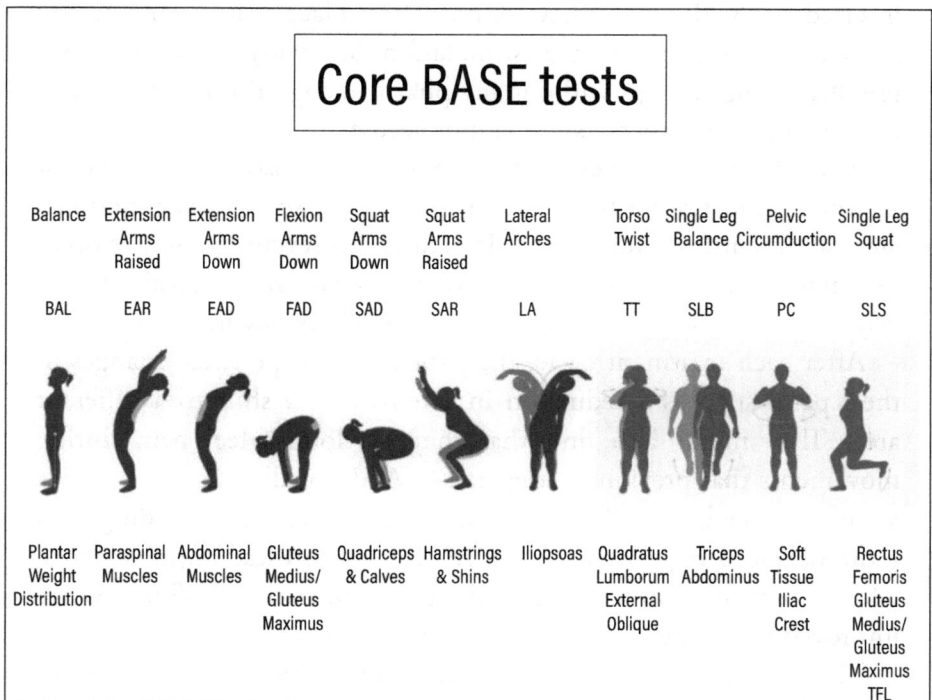

	Balance	Extension Arms Raised	Extension Arms Down	Flexion Arms Down	Squat Arms Down	Squat Arms Raised	Lateral Arches		Torso Twist	Single Leg Balance	Pelvic Circumduction	Single Leg Squat
	BAL	EAR	EAD	FAD	SAD	SAR	LA		TT	SLB	PC	SLS
	Plantar Weight Distribution	Paraspinal Muscles	Abdominal Muscles	Gluteus Medius/ Gluteus Maximus	Quadriceps & Calves	Hamstrings & Shins	Iliopsoas		Quadratus Lumborum External Oblique	Triceps Abdominus	Soft Tissue Iliac Crest	Rectus Femoris Gluteus Medius/ Gluteus Maximus TFL

Core BASE tests

Figure 1. Image created by Dr. Greg Siren for the Anatomic Medicine Foundation.
A painful or restricted movement indicates that the soft tissues shaded areas are most likely to be contributing to the myofascial dysfunction.

When the specific movements are painful or restricted, the myoClinician can identify the soft tissues contributing to myofascial dysfunction. Each BASE test highlights a specific area causing pain, which becomes the target for treatment. This is why the site for treatment is often not at the pain site.

myoActivation treatment

myoActivation treatment uses a fine-gauge hypodermic needle, which is inserted into palpable pain points in the targeted tissues. This releases tight muscles, scars, or thick and tethered fascia. The needles are quickly inserted and withdrawn; they are not left in place as it is done during acupuncture or intramuscular stimulation. Some myoClinicians use a prefilled saline syringe, without any pharmacologically active agent or ingredient, while others use an empty needle.

After treatment, movements and posture are reassessed in cycles of treatment and testing (called catenated cycles) so that dysfunctional areas are identified and treated. If pain is too severe or for any other reason it is not possible to do the movement tests, there is an alternative way of assessing the patient more passively while they lie down.

After each treatment cycle, the patient may experience changes in their pain, such as a reduction in intensity or a shift to a different area. They might also find that they no longer feel pain during movements that previously triggered it. Additionally, they may notice a shift in weight distribution between their feet, often leading to a more balanced or centralized stance. Thanks to these improvements, when repeating movement tests, the myoClinician will often observe improved flexibility and increased range of motion.[4]

The testing and treatment process can be repeated in multiple cycles. This system helps identify each area requiring treatment. If pain is constant or too excruciating to test with movement, the clinician can use an alternative protocol. They will instead assess passively, using observation, palpation, and specific manoeuvres to test for tightness, painful points, and restrictions while the patient is lying down.

"Definitely more limber. It's like day and night."

—myoActivation patient who experienced
decreased pain in their hips and improved balance

Chapter 2: What kinds of pain does myoActivation help?

"This is amazing—you are kidding. This is definitely very different."

—myoActivation patient treated for lower back and upper leg pain

Key points

- myoActivation can treat diverse kinds of pain in different parts of the body.
- Even if the pain has a source you already know about, myoActivation might be able to help.
- The spot where the clinician puts the needle might not always be where you feel pain.
- myoActivation uses movement tests to find the source of pain, but if you can't do them, the clinician can assess you while you're lying down.

Myofascial dysfunction can have widespread effects on the body, making myoActivation a valuable tool for treating numerous conditions. For instance, past injuries and childhood scars can persist as sources of pain and cause movement restrictions for decades. Importantly, experiencing prolonged pain does not imply it is untreatable. It is often possible to alleviate or completely resolve long-standing pain and enhance ranges of motion, even when that pain has been present for many years.

Many patients successfully treated with myoActivation arrived with diagnoses such as spinal stenosis, arthritis, herniated discs, or multiple sclerosis. However, it is important to recognize that myofascial factors may also contribute to the underlying pain experienced with these conditions. So, even with these diagnoses in the background, addressing myofascial components can lead to pain reduction.

Conditions treated by myoActivation

myoActivation can help with:

- Non-specific back pain
- Neck pain, whiplash, wry neck, loss of range of motion in neck movements, or stiffness
- Migraines and various headaches, including tension headache, occipital neuralgia (headache running from the top of the spinal cord to the scalp), and ocular migraine (headache behind the eyes). Most of these ailments are treated by targeting core muscles and deep tension lines in the body.
- Shoulder pain, frozen shoulder, impingement syndrome (shoulder pain from tendons being pinched in the shoulder during movement), rotator cuff injuries, tendonitis (inflammation of a tendon), or general loss of range of motion in the shoulder.
- Hip, knee, leg, or ankle pain
- Arthritis pain
- Temporomandibular joint pain (pain and tenderness in the jaw joints and surrounding muscles), jaw tightness, jaw clicking or opening skew
- Pelvic pain
- Facial and dental pain when no cause can be found by a dentist (it may be referred pain, which is pain felt in a different area of the body than where the actual problem or injury is located)

- Arm or wrist pain, carpal tunnel symptoms, tenosynovitis (inflammation of the tendon sheath), painful thumbs, trigger fingers, early Dupuytren's contractures (thickening of tissue in the palm, causing fingers to curl inward), or epicondylitis (pain and inflammation around the elbow)
- Foot pain, including plantar fasciitis (heel pain caused by the tissue inflammation), pain from bunions, pain from Morton's neuroma (a thickened nerve in the ball of the foot causing pain)
- Leg muscle pain, meralgia paraesthetica (a condition where a nerve in the outer thigh gets compressed, causing numbness, tingling, or burning pain in that area), groin afflictions and strains
- Any painful or tight scars from surgery or previous injuries like burns, road rashes, or accidental cuts
- Tail bone pain or pain on sitting
- Shortness of breath caused by tightness in the chest wall can occur alongside conditions like asthma or other pulmonary diseases. It may also be linked to feelings of anxiety and a heightened adrenaline response, which can make breathing feel even more restricted and uncomfortable.
- Mastectomy scar pain. Due to previous cancer treatment or gender reassignment, these scars may cause restriction over the chest wall, which affects the ability to breathe freely and can restrict shoulder movement or cause pain in the shoulders and neck.
- Non-cardiac chest pain/costochondritis (the inflammation of the cartilage that connects the ribs to the breastbone) or pain over the ribs.
- Abdominal wall pain or tightness, abdominal wall rigidity and dysfunction caused by issues like:
    - Endometriosis,[5] which is a condition where tissue similar to the lining of the uterus grows outside of it, causing pain and sometimes fertility issues.
    - Diverticulitis, which is an infection or inflammation of small pouches in the intestines, causing pain

and digestive problems. If untreated, it can lead to complications like peritonitis, which is a serious infection of the abdominal lining.
- ○ Core muscle strain
- Nerve entrapment syndromes, diabetic neuropathy (nerve damage from high blood sugar)
- Pain in or around any scars resulting from surgeries such as abdominoplasties (tummy tuck), C-sections, and appendectomies (removal of appendix), especially when the surgery occurred at an early age
- Chronic fatigue
- Complex regional pain syndromes (chronic pain conditions that usually affect a limb after injury or surgery) and central sensitization[6] (a condition where the central nervous system becomes overly sensitive to pain)
- Muscles in spasm, or in a constant state of tension
- Spasticity in a muscle (a condition where muscles become stiff and tight, making movement difficult or uncontrollable) due to a central nervous system cause such as multiple sclerosis, cerebral palsy, and stroke. It is possible to reduce the spasticity and tightness for weeks to months at a time, relieving the pain and improving quality of life.
- Spinal pain of musculoskeletal origin

This list is not exhaustive, and each patient living with pain has a unique and different combination of symptoms. Still, it is surprising how many different pain presentations can be helped by releasing myofascial tension.

Example of interconnected pain sources

A common scenario involves patients experiencing constant pain and aches that persist regardless of their posture or position, making it particularly troublesome when trying to sleep. These symptoms can manifest in various sensations, such as tension, toothache-like discomfort, or throbbing, which can worsen at rest or with movement.

The Constant Pain Protocol, developed by the author for patients unable to perform the BASE (movement) tests due to pain intensity, balance issues, or for any other reason, allows for assessment without active movement.

Many of these patients have tried various other treatment approaches with little improvement and often find no lasting relief. It has become clear that when myofascial dysfunction is involved, the source of tension is often far from the site of pain, sometimes in a completely different anatomical region.

For example, tightness in the trapezius muscles (next to the neck) may stem from tension in the abdominal fascia, while neck pain may result from muscles over the sternum pulling on fascia that runs up the sternocleidomastoid muscle (on the side of the neck) muscles, leading to tension at the back of the head and a forward head position. The body is interconnected, and distortions in one area can trigger a range of symptoms elsewhere.

During a visit to their myoClinician, patients can anticipate a comprehensive posture assessment where possible. Treatments may be applied in areas far from where the symptoms are felt, often yielding surprising results.

"It went from hard rock to Jell-O. That's great."

—myoActivation patient when right elbow pain was relieved

Chapter 3: How is myoActivation different from other needling techniques?

*"I hate coming here because I hate needles, but
I [am] also loving coming here."*

—myoActivation patient

- There are other therapies that involve needling, which might seem similar to myoActivation.
- In myoActivation, the spots that are treated are often further away from the place that hurts.
- myoActivation is also different because of the type of needle, what happens with the needle, and what is inside the needle.

    ○ myoActivation uses a hypodermic needle like the ones used in flu shots, which is sharp and thin, to minimize tissue damage.
    ○ The needle is quickly inserted and then removed right away.
    ○ The needle is empty or has a little salt water in it. myoActivation relies on the body's reaction to needling rather than any substance inside the needle.

Overview of common needling techniques

Before we dive into what distinguishes myoActivation, let's start with an overview of some needling techniques.

Intramuscular stimulation (IMS)

IMS, also known as dry needling, treats chronic pain and muscle tightness.[7] It involves inserting thin, sterile acupuncture needles directly into the areas identified as the target for treatment, such as scars or areas of myofascial dysfunction. These needles, with their tapered tips, may be manipulated to cause muscles to twitch and are left in for a short time. Most often, the areas close to the pain are targeted for treatment.

IMS is based on the traditional acupuncture principles but is grounded in Western medicine, considering dermatomes (areas of skin supplied by a specific nerve and its referral area). It aims to stimulate the affected muscles and nerves to promote healing.

In IMS therapy, electricity may be applied to the needles to enhance the treatment's effects. It helps activate the muscles and nerves at the needle site, encouraging them to contract and relax.

Acupuncture

Acupuncture is a traditional Chinese medical practice that involves inserting thin needles into specific points on the body.[8] These points are believed to correspond to energy pathways (meridian lines) that influence various bodily functions. The aim is to release areas where the energy flow is blocked. These needles, which have tapered tips, can be left in for up to forty-five minutes or more and are sometimes manipulated to increase the stimulus. Western-trained acupuncturists often also consider soft tissue dysfunction along anatomic lines and rely less on traditional Chinese practices.

Prolotherapy

Prolotherapy, short for "proliferative therapy," is a medical treatment that stimulates the body's natural healing processes to strengthen injured tissues, such as ligaments and tendons. It involves the injection of a solution, typically a mixture of dextrose (a type of sugar water) and a local anesthetic, into the affected area, near the site of pain or injury.

The injected solution is irritating and triggers a localized inflammatory response. This inflammation prompts the body to send healing cells and nutrients to the area through increased circulation, promoting tissue repair and regeneration. Over time, this process may increase the stability and strength of the injured tissues.

Prolotherapy is often used to address conditions such as joint instability, musculoskeletal injuries, osteoarthritis, and certain types of back pain. It is considered a minimally invasive procedure and is usually performed on an outpatient basis. Multiple sessions of prolotherapy injections may be required to achieve the desired therapeutic effect.[9]

This treatment may also include perineural therapy, which involves injecting a low-dose dextrose solution around irritated nerves to reduce inflammation and pain. It may be combined with hydro-dissection, where fluid is used to separate tissues to target nerve entrapment, which causes discomfort. These approaches use lower, non-irritating doses of dextrose. Their suggested mechanisms include reducing the pain signals in specific sensory nerves by calming their activity.

Platelet-rich plasma (PRP) therapy

PRP therapy involves taking a small sample of the patient's blood and separating the platelets (which help with clotting and healing) and plasma (the liquid part of the blood). These components are rich in growth factors that aid tissue repair. The concentrated platelets and plasma are then injected into the painful or damaged areas to stimulate healing and tissue regeneration.

Key differences with myoActivation

- It focuses on areas for treatment based on the understanding of the patient's indepth injury history.
- Postural assessments and movement tests identify areas that need treatment. myoActivation seldom treats the site where it hurts; this is a key and major difference.
- The needle type that myoActivation therapy utilizes is a common hypodermic needle (like one used for immunizations), which is not left in the body.
- The effect on the tissues differs significantly due to needle type, insertion techniques, and tissue responses compared to other modalities. Specifically, the use of cutting-tip needles in myoActivation provides a minimally traumatic stimulus, triggering a spinal reflex, inducing muscle relaxation, as well as releasing tension in the fascia.
- Some myoActivation clinicians may use a syringe filled with saline, but this is free of any irritants or pharmacologically active chemicals.
- Electricity is not applied to the needles as may happen in IMS.

By focusing on the unique needs of each patient and using specific assessment methods, myoActivation provides a targeted, low-impact approach to pain management. Its emphasis on indirect treatment sites, reliance on body responses, and minimally invasive approach set it apart from other needling methods.

"My life is so different without the migraines: I have more energy and can do more activities. I am so excited."

—myoActivation patient

Chapter 4: How does myoActivation work?

"My life has changed since I started treatment,
my gait is less jerky, and more fluid and I can move better."

—myoActivation patient with multiple sclerosis

myoActivation works by targeting three key tissue types: scars, muscles, and fascia. The treatment helps release tight areas, or "knots," in these tissues, helping to reduce pain and improving movement. By loosening muscles and fascia, myoActivation relieves tension and reduces the pulling on surrounding joints and structures. This release helps improve flexibility, decreases pressure on joints, and promotes better overall function throughout the body.

What happens to the tissues?

Key points

- Needling works on three types of tissues: scars, tight muscles, and problems with the fascia.
- Needling causes scars to reheal a little less tightly, removing pressure on your body.

- Needling makes tight muscles relax due to a reflex (an automatic reaction in the nervous system).
- It also relaxes the fascial tissues and helps them move smoothly over each other.
- Overall, myoActivation decreases pain, improves flexibility, and supports ease of movement.
- myoActivation can also help the body feel calmer when it has less tension.
- Reduced tension and pain improves mental health.
- When tissues are less tight, blood flow also improves.

The various tissue types targeted by myoActivation can each feel different and have a unique response to needling. Usually, the target of treatment is one of three tissues:

- Scars
- Muscles
- Fascia

Needling can effectively address the effects of scar tissue, tight muscles, and fascial components of pain and dysfunction.[10] As a result, many patients experience improved mobility, reduced pain, and enhanced overall function.[11]

Here is an overview of what happens in the various tissues during needling:

Scars

When needling scars, a cutting-tip needle simulates the effect of a microblade. This process divides the fibres in the scar, facilitates remodelling, and promotes maturation of the scar through a new or resumed healing response. Because a small-gauge needle is used, the body does not have to heal an entire wound.[12] Later in this chapter, more detailed information on scar release and its global effects is provided.

It could be beneficial to take a "before" photo of any major scars and again after undergoing myoActivation treatment, as scar remodelling can dramatically improve the cosmetic appearance. This improvement may include a lighter appearance, resulting in a scar that is flatter, less tight or tethered to the underlying tissues.

Scar tissue affects the surrounding fascia, which has a far-reaching impact, distorting the connective tissue surrounding and supporting the whole body.

Muscles

Trigger points, or "knots," are small, tight areas of muscle that can cause pain[13] and even send pain to other areas of the body. When a hypodermic (cutting-tip) needle is inserted into a contracted muscle, it causes a protective spinal reflex to fire, causing the muscle to relax.[14] This may be felt as a "twitch." The reflex causes a reset of the muscle fibres, releasing tension and reducing pain.[15]

Tight muscles can exert pressure on joints, interfering with their function and causing pain in the joint. For example, if the quadricep muscles are tight, they can pull on the patella (kneecap), compressing it and increasing pressure on the knee joint. This can lead to knee pain and, over time, may accelerate joint degeneration. Even individuals with hypermobility (joints that can move beyond the typical range of motion) can experience tightness in their muscles.

Fascia

During myoActivation, the fascia (the body-wide connective tissue) is impacted. The needles are inserted into tight or restricted areas, which can feel like painful, knotted points made up of muscle and fascia. This tightness can extend throughout the fascia itself, and releasing this tension can have a global effect on function and pain.

Releasing one area can alleviate tension in the connected fascial pathways far away from the site of release through myofascial chains. This provides not only local pain relief but also in the affected fascial regions.

Adhesions or restrictions within the fascia hinder the natural gliding and sliding of fascial layers. Treating these improves mobility and allows for smoother movement between the planes of fascial layers.

Releasing tight areas reduces pressure and tension, facilitating better microcirculation. This improved blood flow supports tissue healing, aids nutrient delivery, and removes waste.[16]

Other effects of needling

Needling techniques can also have multiple whole-body effects, including reduced stress hormone levels,[17] vascular effects (improved circulation and oxygenation), and effects on the central and peripheral nervous system. In turn, reduced stress improves emotional regulation, and a reduction in chronic pain can decrease depressive symptoms.[18] As a result, general well-being is improved.

Being able to move better and with less or no pain allows for more activity, which increases production of endorphins (the happy hormone),[19] and this promotes a sense of positivity and hope.[20]

> *"I'm so grateful to be here. It's hard to imagine in this short amount of time, there has been a difference."*

—myoActivation patient, referring to the reduction in pain and tension in the calves and upper legs after the first treatment

Chapter 5: Can scars cause pain?

*"That's bizarre. I am feeling like my foot just dropped [relaxed].
I want to cry because I have never not felt tension in my body."*
—myoActivation patient

Key points

- A scar creates tension in your skin and fascial tissue.
- Tension in one spot can pull on other tissues.
- Pain from a scar can appear far away from the scar itself.
- Needling breaks down the scar, so it pulls less on the skin and fascial tissue, easing pain and improving blood flow.
- The healing process can also cause scars to look less red or flatter against the skin. If you're having a scar treated, you should take a picture before treatment to compare it to the result afterward.
- Scar needling can take multiple sessions to remodel the scar tissue.

Part of the myoActivation assessment is focused on identifying scar tissue on the skin. The skin, which is the largest organ of the body, connects to deeper fascia, muscles, and bones through superficial fascia. Additionally, skin is richly supplied with nerves that connect to the central nervous system. Scars—from surgery, burns, or injuries—can disrupt these connections and lead to myofascial dysfunctions.

When the skin structure is disrupted (for instance, through surgery), its structure changes and scars form, affecting how skin functions and communicates with other body parts.[21] This is why, during the myoActivation assessment, patients are asked about previous surgeries, burns, broken bones, cuts, traumatic events, or any other significant injuries.

Scars greatly impact how tension distributes within the body, as the affected tissues may not stretch or move as they should. Other areas must then compensate for this added resistance instead of stretching normally or gliding over each other.

For example, abdominal scars create tension in the front of the body, forcing back muscles to work harder to maintain posture.[22] This extra effort puts pressure on the surrounding bones and discs, affects soft tissues, joints, and nerves, and causes symptoms such as back pain. Interestingly, although the pain may be felt in the back, the root cause often originates from issues occurring in the front of the body where the scar is located.

The tension from scars isn't limited to just one area. For instance, tension from abdominal scars can also spread and cause tightness in the neck and shoulders. This example highlights how scars, regardless of their size, age, origin, or apparent significance, can affect the body by creating tension along fascial lines. This tension often leads to pain or restricted movement in both local and distant areas. Even tiny scars, like chickenpox marks, can have a significant effect. Releasing tension in the fascia inside and around these scars can improve movement and reduce pain.

Burn scars are especially important to consider because they can cause the skin and tissues to contract. But even old burn scars can respond well to needling.[23] Apart from enhancing aesthetics by reducing redness, needling can effectively diminish tension. This process facilitates tissue remodelling and increases movement and flexibility.

Scar release with needling is a therapeutic technique used to improve the function and state of the tissue in and underneath scars from surgeries and/or trauma.[24] Through needling, controlled micro-injuries are created in the scar tissue, which helps stimulate the body's natural healing response and the scars are remodelled.

The goal in needling scars is to break up collagen, adhesions, and restrictions. This improves tissue mobility and flexibility, reduces pain, and restores function.

Though improving how a scar looks isn't the primary goal, it can be fascinating to see how scars can remodel after needling. People often do not like to look at their scars, making it hard to remember how they looked before the treatment. For this reason, taking a photo of any scars before they are treated is recommended so that the change can be fully appreciated.

The effects of scar release with needling

Controlled micro-injury and inflammation

When the needle makes tiny cuts in the scar tissue, these micro-injuries trigger a localized inflammatory response. Inflammation is essential to the healing process as it increases blood flow, delivering nutrients, growth factors, and immune cells to the area.[25]

Collagen remodelling

The inflammatory response initiates the release of growth factors, particularly the transforming growth factor beta (TGF-beta). This growth factor plays a crucial role in collagen production and remodelling, promoting capillaries' growth, enhancing blood supply and facilitating tissue repair and regeneration.

Scar tissue, which is typically dense and fibrous, often limits movement and causes discomfort. However, with needling and collagen remodelling, the scar tissue transforms. It becomes softer, more elastic, and less tightly bound to underlying structures. As a result, individuals undergoing myoActivation treatment experience improved mobility and pain reduction in local and distal areas.[26]

Fascia release

Scar tissue can also affect the surrounding fascia. Needling helps release tension and adhesions that form in the fascial layers, reducing restrictions and improving overall tissue function.

Reduced nerve compression

Scar tissue can entrap or compress nerves, leading to pain or various symptoms (such as numbness, tingling, cold sensations, or burning sensation). Scar release techniques can alleviate nerve compression, reducing these symptoms.

Improved circulation and lymph flow

Scars can compress local capillaries, the larger blood vessels, and the lymphatic system, which help maintain fluid balance, remove waste, and fight infections. Needling the scar releases tissue compression over the blood vessels and lymphatic system. This brings additional nutrients and oxygen to the area, as well as improves waste removal, and further supports the healing process and tissue regeneration.

Reducing the tension within scars causes a reduction in pain, improved tissue mobility and restored function.

It is important to note that scar release with needling should be performed by trained professionals who understand the anatomy of the area and have experience with the procedure. Depending on the tightness and type of scar, multiple sessions may be needed to achieve the desired results.

"Went in and I could hardly stand or move my head, fifteen minutes of treatment, and I was good to go."
—Google review of the myoClinic Brentwood Bay

Chapter 6: Why do muscles hurt?

"Amazing treatments of my muscles that felt like rock hard;
she simply popped a tiny needle in it, and poof, no longer
a tough muscle soft and relaxed without more meds! I now
look forward to my next session in January 2024."

—Google review of the myoClinic Brentwood Bay

Key points

- Muscles can become stiff or sore if you overwork them or hold them in the same position for a long time.
- There are also neurological conditions like multiple sclerosis and Parkinson's disease that cause tight muscles.
- Tight muscles can be released with myoActivation.
- myoActivation can't cure a neurological condition, but it can help make the symptoms easier to live with.

Several mechanisms can cause muscles to feel tight and sore. For instance, when a muscle is subjected to intense activity, activity it is not used to, or as a result of some underlying neurological (nerve) conditions, it can get caught in a state called hypertonicity.[27] Hypertonicity refers to a muscle contracting more than usual and staying engaged, unable to relax. The resulting tightness causes tension and pain and is often tender when pressed on.

Muscle fibres in a contracted state can experience reduced blood flow and oxygen supply, causing the buildup of waste products like lactic acid.[28] This buildup of metabolites (the by-products of normal metabolic processes) triggers pain and discomfort. Also, micro-tears in the muscle fibres, especially when the activity is new or intense, contribute to the soreness. Consequently, tightness can affect the range of motion and put pressure on joints, affecting how the body functions and moves.

Sometimes, maintaining a sedentary posture for an extended period of time can cause contractions or shortening of muscles. If, for example, a person always sits leaning toward one arm of their favourite couch, especially over prolonged periods of time, the repetitiveness of this posture can cause muscles to stiffen or shorten.[29] They may feel stiff and/or sore when they finally get up.

Another issue can be tight core (abdominal) musculature. Tight muscles in the core can impact balance, walking, and other physical activities.[30]

There are also neurological causes for muscles being rigid, tight, or spastic (continuously tight and rigid muscles), such as:

- stroke
- multiple sclerosis
- Parkinson's disease
- nerve damage
- amyotrophic lateral sclerosis (also known as motor neurone disease or Lou Gehrig's disease)

This is not an exhaustive list, but releasing tight muscles, fascia, or scars can improve the range of motion and reduce pain in many conditions. Releasing the myofascial tissues contributing to muscle tightness does not cure the neurological condition or an underlying disease process but can help improve quality of life.

"This is mind-blowing."

—myoActivation patient after first treatment for migraine at the myoClinic Brentwood Bay; the migraine lifted during treatment

Chapter 7: What is the fascial system?

*"I don't think it [the leg and hip joint] has
moved that much since I was a kid."*

—this myoActivation patient gained a greater
range of movement after treatment

Key points

- Fascia is a tissue network like a bodysuit that surrounds and connects all parts of your body. It has a lot of nerve endings, like your skin.
- The fascial system provides structure, support, and protection to other parts of your body. It also helps tissues move over each other.
- Fascia is adaptable and responds to stress and movement.
- Myofascial dysfunction is when your muscles and the fascia connected to them aren't working correctly. Because fascia keeps your body balanced, if it gets pulled out of place, becomes dry, or gets stuck together, it can cause problems all over your body.
- Myofascial dysfunction can hurt and make it hard to move.

A group of international scientists published the following definition of the fascial system in the *Journal of Bodywork and Movement Therapies*:

The fascial system consists of the three-dimensional continuum of soft, collagen containing loose and dense fibrous connective tissues that permeate the body. It incorporates elements such as adipose tissue [body fat], adventitiae [outer layers of blood vessels] and neurovascular sheaths [protective coverings for nerves and blood vessels], aponeuroses [flat sheets of connective tissue that connect muscles], deep and superficial fasciae, epineurium [outer covering of nerves], joint capsules, ligaments, membranes, meninges [protective layers covering the brain and spinal cord], myofascial expansions [extensions of muscle connective tissue], periostea [outer layers of bones], retinacula [bands of connective tissue that hold tendons in place], septa [dividing walls between tissues], tendons, visceral fasciae [connective tissue around internal organs], and all the intramuscular and intermuscular connective tissues including endo-/peri-/epimysium [layers of connective tissue within muscles]. The fascial system surrounds, interweaves between, and interpenetrates all organs, muscles, bones, and nerve fibres, endowing the body with a functional structure, and providing an environment that enables all body systems to operate in an integrated manner. [31]

In other words, fascia is a specialized tissue that surrounds and interconnects throughout the human body, through muscles, over joints, bones, organs, nerves, and blood vessels. It wraps around and weaves through all tissues in the body, and it plays a significant role in movement and maintaining overall health and well-being.

To reiterate, fascia holds everything in place and is pivotal in helping our muscles, joints, and organs to glide smoothly over each other during movement. Furthermore, not only does fascia provide structural support and protection, like scaffolding, but it is also an important sensory organ, sending information to the brain about our position as well as pain in our body.

Fascia is also like the structure in an orange, the white pith-like casing immediately under the orange skin or rind. Oranges are divided into segments, and if one were to open an individual segment, tiny pockets of juice encased by a fascial layer would be noticed. The fascia keeps the tiny orange pockets all together in an organized structure.

Fascia consists of a fibre matrix, ground substance, and cells. The fibres consist of collagen and elastin. They are incredibly strong and flexible and contain several cell types that maintain them.[32] For instance, fasciacytes (specific cells in fascia) produce the hyaluronan-rich extracellular matrix[33] that promotes various tissues' ability to slide and glide over each other during movement. It also serves as a transport system for water and electrolytes aided by the pumping action of muscular contraction.

Fascia works as a tension network through the body, connecting localized muscles with groups that work further away to keep the body balanced.[34] Mechanical forces are generated and pass through this tension network when we move. The balance in our bodies that our fascia maintains is called tensional integrity or "tensegrity."

Our bodily structures and movements are stabilized by this balance between tension (stretching forces) and compression (pushing forces) to allow for efficient movement and load-bearing capacity. Therefore, disturbances or imbalances in one area of the fascial system, for instance, from injuries, scars, or surgeries,[35] can have repercussions throughout the body, potentially leading to pain, restrictions, or functional limitations throughout.[36]

Fascia dynamically remodels itself in reaction to movement patterns, physical activities, and injuries. This adaptability is crucial to how the body responds to different demands and stresses.[37] It is also why myoClinicians ask patients about their complete history of injuries to the body, including competitive sports and activities. Each activity places a unique set of demands on the body and may contribute to the pain symptoms.

When subjected to repeated stress and tension, fascia adapts in density or thickness as it produces more collagen, rearranges its fibres, and becomes more or less elastic.[38] These changes can lead to either positive or negative effects on the body. For example, regular exercise and movement that promotes healthy fascial plasticity results in improved flexibility, better tissue resilience, and enhanced athletic performance. In contrast, lengthy periods of immobility due to a severe illness, a sedentary lifestyle, or moving in ways that strain the body (called poor movement patterns) may lead to negative changes, such as limited range of motion and a higher risk of injury.

You could also imagine fascia as a bodysuit or onesie. If this suit is distorted by tight muscles or scar tissue, it affects how the whole body functions. Research by a group of scientists from the Academic Medical Centre in the Netherlands[39] showed that 37 percent of muscles connect to the fascial layers rather than directly to the bone. So, when muscles are too tight, they pull on the fascial system in different directions.

When fascia is relatively dry, it becomes inflexible, doesn't move easily, and looks and feels like a gristle. Healthy, hydrated fascia is soft, flexible, and glides easily. Movement helps pump fluids through the layers, keeping the tissue flexible and lubricated. When you sit for a long time, things stagnate, making it harder to move, which can feel stiff, achy, or uncomfortable. In short, fascia is like a washcloth—soft and flexible when wet but becomes rigid when it dries out.

Fascia is also highly innervated, which means it has many nerve endings that send signals about position, temperature, pressure, touch, and pain. Some studies suggest that pain from fascia can be more intense than muscle pain and often feel like stabbing, stinging, or irritating, while muscle pain tends to feel more like a dull ache.[40] Since fascia wraps around many different types of tissues, it's common to experience more than one type of pain at the same time.

Types of fascia

Each type of fascia has a unique location and function. Together, these types of fascia play a crucial role in the structure and function of our bodies and act as a complex sensory system. Let's explore the four types of fascia.

Superficial fascia

Superficial fascia is located just beneath the skin and is composed of loose connective tissue, fat cells, blood vessels, and many nerves. Its thickness varies in different parts of the body. Its primary roles are to provide insulation, cushioning, and support for the skin, allowing it to move freely over the tissues underneath.

Deep fascia

Deep fascia is a dense, fibrous tissue that surrounds and separates muscles and muscle groups, providing support and helping keep them in place. It forms strong sheets that help transmit the forces generated by muscle contractions to other, more distant parts of the body. Deep fascia also creates compartments around muscles, which helps with movement by enhancing the power and efficiency of muscle contractions.

This type of fascia forms a continuous network around muscles, often extending across and through multiple muscle groups. For example, tightness or scarring in the abdominal area from muscle strain or surgery can cause shoulder muscle strain and dysfunction and limit shoulder movement range due to the fascial connections.

Visceral fascia

Visceral fascia covers and supports organs in the chest and abdominal cavities. The term "visceral" refers to the internal organs, so this type of fascia surrounds and protects organs like the lungs (visceral pleura), heart (visceral pericardium) and abdominal organs (visceral peritoneum). It helps these organs move smoothly and prevents friction during natural processes like breathing or digestion. For example, as the lungs expand and contract, the visceral fascia helps reduce friction between the lungs and chest wall, making it easier to breathe.

Periosteum

The periosteum is a thick, fibrous membrane covering the bones' outer surface. It is essential for bone growth, repair, and providing nutrition. This membrane contains blood vessels, nerves, and cells involved in bone formation and remodelling. In addition to nourishing bones, the periosteum is a critical attachment point for ligaments and tendons, which helps with stability and movement. The periosteum covers all bones, except at the joints where the articular cartilage (smooth, protective tissue) covers the bone surfaces.

Myofascial dysfunction (MFD)

Myofascial dysfunction describes the muscles and fascia not working correctly. When fascia becomes tight or inflamed, it can restrict movement and cause pain. This can happen due to muscles staying contracted for extended periods or scar tissue, limiting the ability of tissues to glide smoothly.[41] As a result, the system becomes stuck, leading to restricted movement, discomfort, and unusual sensations in the body.

MFD has wide-ranging effects. Tight muscles in one area can influence the entire body through fascial connections.[42] Pain in one spot may be caused by dysfunction in distant, seemingly unrelated areas—a concept called regional interdependence.

Tightness in the body can also affect the autonomic nervous system, which controls internal functions like circulation, blood pressure, and digestion. This can have a profound effect on emotional regulation as well.[43]

Causes and treatment of MFD

Various factors can cause fascia to become tight, restricted (as in skin creases or scars), or overly sensitive. This includes muscle overuse, previous injuries, poor posture, and emotional stress.[44] Tight areas of muscle, called trigger points, and denser areas of fascia contribute to chronic pain, movement limitations, and posture problems. Fascial density also creates tension around joints, further limiting movement and causing discomfort. MFD can start at an early age and persist for years, but it is treatable.

Anatomical distortions in the fascia can have significant consequences. Because fascia forms a continuous, interconnected network throughout the body, disruptions in one area can affect distant areas, leading to pain in seemingly unrelated regions.[45] This comes back to a basic principle of myoActivation that the site of pain is not necessarily the true source of pain.

Understanding fascia's interconnected nature helps explain why disturbances in this network contribute to various pain problems. It emphasizes the importance of viewing the body as a 3-D interconnected structure.

MFD can be treated through approaches like myoActivation, stretching, massage, physical therapy, yoga, dry needling, and cortisone injections.

Sometimes, conditions like arthritis or a herniated disc might be diagnosed, but MFD may also be contributing by creating tension and pressure on joints, nerves, and soft tissues. Releasing these tight areas can significantly reduce chronic pain and tension, even if imaging still shows signs of arthritis or disc herniation. Many chronic pain conditions have myofascial components, regardless of the diagnosis.

MFD distorts the body's intricate fascial network, leading to pain and restricted movement. Understanding the interconnectedness of fascia and the treatment options available can help address these issues and improve well-being.

"It feels like night and day but still feels a bit tight to left."

—myoActivation patient referred for pain
and difficulty rotating the spine

Chapter 8: What to expect during myoActivation treatment?

"That's amazing; it feels like it's unwinding; it feels a lot better; it's a good over 90 percent better—it's like magic."

—myoActivation patient who presented with severe lower back pain

The first appointment

Key points

- Your first appointment at a myoActivation clinic will involve talking about your medical history, an assessment of your posture, and some movement tests.
- The clinician will ask you about any surgeries, accidents, scars, or broken bones you've had in your life. They will also ask about medications you've taken and if you played competitive sports as a child.
- The purpose of this appointment is to determine where your pain is coming from.
- If you can't do the movement tests because they hurt too much, the clinician can use a different assessment that will take place while you're lying down. Once your pain improves, then you can try the movement tests again.

- Wear loose, comfortable clothes that allow your arms and legs to be easily seen during your appointment. If you have long hair, please tie it back to help the clinician examine any scars and muscle knots.

The first visit will be a consultation with a myoActivation clinician (myoClinician), lasting between thirty and sixty minutes, depending on the clinic. It often includes the first myoActivation treatment.

Patients are advised to wear loose, comfortable clothes that expose their arms and legs—shorts, a skirt, a T-shirt, or a tank top—and to tie back long hair to allow the clinician to examine their shoulders and neck.

The initial part of the appointment focuses on gathering a detailed medical history, called a timeline of lifetime traumas (TiLT). TiLT includes questions about previous surgeries, accidents, fractures, scars and participation in competitive sports, especially during childhood. These prior injuries can contribute to the current array of symptoms. The discussion also covers medication history, including the use of blood thinners or immune suppressants. Additionally, any concerns or questions, such as needle aversion, will be addressed.

Next, a posture assessment is done in a relaxed standing pose. This is followed by a series of specific movement tests known as BASE (biomechanical assessment and symmetry evaluation), designed to identify asymmetries, assess ranges of movement, and focus on movements that cause the most pain or restriction. The BASE tests help identify which tissues are involved in the symptoms. Any movement that causes discomfort, tightness, or restriction guides the myoClinician to assess scars and painful spots in the muscles or fascia in that specific area.

It's important to note that the source of dysfunction is often not where the pain is felt or perceived.

When a patient arrives feeling good, subtle signs like limited range of motion or mild discomfort during stretching may still indicate tissue dysfunction. For patients unable to perform movement tests due to severe pain or disability, the myoClinician can perform a passive assessment while the patient is lying down. Once the pain improves, the standard movement tests can be reintroduced to find any remaining areas of dysfunction.

myoActivation Treatment

Key points

- myoActivation treatment involves inserting a thin, sharp needle into specific areas under the skin.
- These areas may be muscle knots, scars, or places where the fascia is misaligned.
- The needle might not be inserted directly where the pain is felt.
- You may feel a pinch, and nearby muscles may twitch, shift, or ache.
- Those sensations can sometimes spread to the other parts of the body.
- Needling can sometimes trigger surprising emotions or old memories.
- If you're in a lot of pain or are afraid of needles, a slow treatment approach with just one or two needles can still help.

The next step is palpation and treatment after the posture assessment and movement tests are completed. This involves using hypodermic needles to release targeted tissues. The needle is inserted and withdrawn quickly—it is never left in the tissue, unlike acupuncture or IMS (intramuscular stimulation).

A prefilled 3-ml (about 0.1 oz) syringe, containing less than a teaspoon of sterile salt water and with no other ingredients, is sometimes used during treatment. Other clinics may do dry needling or use an empty syringe. The effects and outcomes are the same regardless of which method is used.

Often, patients feel a muscle twitch more than the actual needle sensation. A muscle twitch is not necessary for the treatment to be effective. Some patients describe a brief electrical feeling or a shooting sensation as the tissues respond to the needling.

During the first visit, a treatment trial helps introduce the sensation of needling and monitors how the body responds. Some changes can be immediate as muscles twitch and release. While this sensation can be surprising, it is often simultaneously relieving. Posture and movements are reassessed in cycles of test, treat, and retest to direct treatment and track changes.

During and after treatment, patients may notice changes in pain (either reduced or relocated), improved balance, or feeling "lighter." Some may also experience an emotional release, such as tearfulness, as memories of past injuries or surgeries resurface. This phenomenon supports the idea that myofascial tissues may store memories of past physical trauma,[46] and releasing them can be emotionally therapeutic.

Depending on the severity of the pain or response to treatment, there may only be one test-treat-retest cycle during the appointment. However, when possible, several cycles may be performed. If the first area is treated, pain or movement issues may shift to another area, guiding further treatment—this process is sometimes compared to peeling back layers of an onion, as dysfunction is resolved layer by layer.

There may be days when the patient feels more sensitive or would prefer to limit treatment cycles or target areas. This is entirely acceptable. Even a minimal number of needles can provide significant benefits and contribute to the journey toward healing.

Patients who are afraid of needles or have hypersensitivity may only tolerate one or two injection sites per treatment session and may require more sessions spread out over time to address all their myofascial issues. This approach of minimal treatment is also recommended for patients with fibromyalgia to reduce the risk of experiencing a pain flare-up after needling.

As patients experience the benefits of myoActivation, their nervous system usually becomes more relaxed, allowing them to tolerate more needles in future sessions. Distraction techniques, such as breathing techniques, squeezing stress balls, or listening to music, can also help reduce discomfort during the procedure. These are especially important for children and youth to make visits more pleasant.

When patients know what to expect, they feel more comfortable, more informed, and less anxious about the treatment.

What will I feel during treatment?

Needle insertion sensations

- **An initial prick or pinch:** When the needle is first inserted, there may be a quick, sharp sensation similar to a pinch or a mosquito bite. This is the initial penetration of the skin and muscle and is usually mild and brief.
- **Local twitch response:** A common response to needling is a "twitch response," which feels like a sudden, involuntary muscle contraction or vibration. While it may be surprising, it is a beneficial part of the procedure that helps release tension and improve blood flow. This sensation can follow the direction of the muscles or fascia and may sometimes briefly shoot in other directions. It is often accompanied by a sensation of release, warmth, tingling, and/or relief.
- **Aching or dull pain:** During and after needle insertion, you may feel a brief aching or dull pain, like post-workout fatigue in the muscle. This is normal and a good sign, but let the myoClinician know if the pain becomes too uncomfortable.

Other sensations

- **Burning or warmth:** Some patients report a burning or warm sensation at the insertion site. This is temporary and may suggest mild bruising. Applying a little pressure can help ease the sensation and prevent bruising.

- **Radiating sensations:** These sensations may extend from the insertion point to other body parts. For instance, a release in the thigh muscles might be felt in the toe or the foot on the same side. This is common and indicates that the tension source has been released, reducing referred pain. Referred pain is felt in one area of the body but originates elsewhere. Patients often describe the feeling as "electrical," followed by a sensation of relief and ease.

Emotional release

- **Emotional responses:** Some areas carry an emotional component, which may be linked to past trauma. When treated, patients may feel tearful, angry, sad or remember a traumatic event. Sometimes the emotion can be accompanied by flashbacks of images, memories, scents, or sounds. This release can be surprising or unsettling, but it is normal. On occasion, patients can connect this response to a specific event or trauma, while at other times, there is no apparent reason for the emotional response.
- These reactions are not unusual and are viewed as a positive shift in the nervous system, often leading to reduced pain and improved function. If you experience this reaction, taking time for self-care—journaling, breathing exercises, meditation—or consulting a trauma-informed counsellor can help process any resurfaced emotions.

What to expect after the appointment?

Key points

- After the appointment, you may feel sore and tired for a few days. That's normal. Rest and drink plenty of water. The needle site may bruise, and the pain might move to another spot, which is also normal.
- After the initial soreness goes away, you should start to feel the benefits of the treatment, with less pain and easier movement.
- If a muscle cramps up after the appointment, you should tell your clinician because it may need more treatment to release fully.
- If you have an autoimmune condition or a heightened pain sensitivity, you may experience a pain flare-up lasting for a few days. myoActivation can still help you, but the treatment may need to proceed gradually.
- If you have trouble breathing or a fever, tell your clinician immediately or contact your doctor.

What to expect after each appointment

- **Improvement in symptoms:** myoActivation aims to reduce pain and improve function.
- **Change in pain site:** If pain moves to a new area, this is a positive sign, even if it feels uncomfortable initially.
- **Soreness:** Mild soreness at the treatment sites is common and usually subsides in a day or two after treatment. Over-the-counter medication can help if needed.
- **Bruising:** Mild bruising may occasionally occur at the injection site. Pressing on the bruise for one minute can limit its size.

Bruising usually clears up within two weeks, though it may feel tender.

- **Fatigue:** Feeling tired after treatment is normal. Rest, drink enough fluids, and give your body time to recover.
- **Cramping:** Let your myoClinician know if you experience cramping, as it may mean that there was a partial release, and additional treatment is needed to fully release the muscle in the cramping area.
- **Pain flare-ups:** In a small number of cases—especially for patients with pre-existing heightened pain sensation or autoimmune diseases—a temporary pain flare-up may occur, lasting three to five days, or in exceedingly rare cases, a few weeks. If this happens, the treatment is customized with fewer needles and more recovery time between sessions while still providing benefits like reduced tension and increased mobility.
- **Rare side effects:**
  - **Pneumothorax:** Pneumothorax occurs when air enters the space around the lungs, known as the pleural space. This is a particularly rare side effect that can happen after needling in areas near the chest. A pneumothorax feels like pressure in the chest, a feeling of not being able to take a full breath or shortness of breath. Although pneumothorax is rare, it can require assessment by a medical professional. The small amount of air involved usually gets absorbed by the body naturally over a few days, and needing a procedure like a chest drain (to resolve pneumothorax) is rare. If you experience these symptoms, contact your clinician or go to the emergency department.
  - **Infection:** Infection risk around the needle entry site is extremely low due to the use of sterile needles and extra precautions taken in immune-compromised patients. However, it is important to let your myoClinician know if you are prone to skin infections or have a compromised immune system. Typical

post-treatment effects include mild redness, tenderness, and occasional bruising. These usually resolve within a day or two. You should inform your myoClinician if you notice increasing pain, heat, swelling, fever, or worsening symptoms.

Follow-up treatments typically last between ten and thirty minutes, but they can be longer depending on how a clinic runs its appointments and schedule. Follow-up visits are shorter than the initial consultation. The discomfort of needling is tolerated well, with most patients finding the eventual benefits worth any minor discomfort from needling compared to their usual pain.

Each myoClinician may have a slightly different approach to the follow-up routine. For example, at the myoClinic Brentwood Bay, two follow-up appointments (fifteen minutes each) are scheduled a week apart after the initial thirty-minute consultation. These three initial appointments are pre-booked to secure time slots before the schedule fills up, but adjustments can be made to accommodate personal needs.

Each myoClinician may tailor appointment durations and schedules to suit the specific patient profile they serve.

Follow up appointments

Key points

- At your next appointment, your clinician will ask you to talk about how you felt after the treatment and if your pain has changed.
- Please keep track of how you feel the week after your appointment; this information helps your clinician decide on the next steps.
- If you are worried about forgetting, consider keeping a pain journal (an example is provided at the end of Chapter 10), or you can track in any way that works for you.

- At each appointment, your clinician will discuss aftercare instructions. Following these instructions will make treatment more effective.
- If you have upcoming intense physical tasks, like building a deck or moving furniture, your clinician may suggest postponing your appointment to avoid extra stress on your body.
- Between appointments, take short breaks every fifteen minutes if you are sitting, get up and stretch, or take a quick rest if you are moving around.
- The first three appointments will be close together, and it's best to avoid too much strenuous physical activity during this time. Later, appointments will be spaced out about a month apart, and you can start gradually increasing physical activities again.

At follow-up appointments, questions might include:

- How did your body respond to the treatment?
- How sore, tired, or achy did you feel?
- Did you have any emotional responses?
- Did you notice changes in the character or location of your pain?
- Has there been a change in what causes pain?
- Have you noticed any other changes, perhaps in sleep, energy levels, or range of movement?
- Has your pain changed from being constant to intermittent, or vice versa?
- If you experience migraines, did they change in intensity, location, duration, associated symptoms, or medication needed?
- What are you most aware of currently (because pain can move as various areas are released)?

Posture and movement checks

Posture and movement tests will be briefly rechecked during each follow-up visit based on the current symptoms. Patients will undergo repeated cycles of movement testing, treatment of problem areas, and retesting until the desired result is achieved.

Aftercare instructions

Aftercare instructions will be provided in Chapter 10 and during appointments, and any questions can be addressed. Following the aftercare instructions can minimize the need for further treatment on the same tissues, support the treatment's effectiveness, and speed up recovery.

Duration and frequency

On average, most patients need between three and eight sessions to address multiple sources of myofascial dysfunction. Recovery time after the needling technique is very individual and can change from one treatment session to the next. Some people no longer feel changes after twenty-four hours; others can take a week or a few weeks for the changes to stabilize. On average, the body stabilizes within three to five days.

Tracking progress

Checking in with your body during the week after treatment and noticing any changes can be helpful. If you find this difficult, using a pain journal (see Chapter 10) can help track without focusing all attention on pain. Instead, it helps to simply note the area and intensity of any sensations felt during the day.

Body awareness and communication

Patients are encouraged to share their experiences with their myoClinician after treatment. Some may find it helpful to keep a journal or make notes about after-effects—such as fatigue, achiness, the duration of these effects, and any changes in sensations or function. While some bruising is normal, discuss any concerns with your clinician.

Remembering how you felt weeks ago can be difficult, so simple notes can offer a big-picture view of progress. Sometimes, sensations may shift to different areas, which is a good prognostic sign, but may initially feel uncomfortable. Shifts in body tension can cause achiness because the fascia is richly connected to sensory nerves, and these changes may be complex for the body to interpret.[47]

Finally, report any new injuries, falls, or other physical traumas between treatments, as these can strain tissues in recovery. For example, a fall or strenuous activities like building a deck over the weekend shortly after a needling treatment may delay healing and reduce the benefit of treatment.

Mindful recovery

After treatment, being gentle with your body allows it to reset, restore function, and promote healing. If you have pressing tasks involving high-strain activities shortly after appointments, consider rescheduling your treatment or task to allow yourself some recovery time.

If you keep doing things that strain your body or cause stiffness, you will need treatment again. For example, if hip flexors are treated and you spend hours sitting, the hip flexors will shorten and tighten again.

Releasing the tense soft tissues is only one part of the process toward a better quality of life. The other involves changing the habits that contributed to causing the strain and tension in the first place. Postures or activities that caused strain and tension before may lead to pain again if they remain unchanged.

The goal after treatment is to slowly build up stamina and maintain flexibility. Gentle strengthening, physiotherapy, stretching, and massage can extend the benefits of myoActivation. Activities can be gradually increased to build stamina to support a more functional lifestyle with less pain.

Best aftercare practices

Aim to change your posture every ten to fifteen minutes during the first few days after treatment. For example, if sitting, stand up every fifteen minutes to gently stretch or take a short walk intermittently; if standing, sit for a moment to relax. Avoid holding any one posture for too long.

Communication with your myoClinician

Throughout the procedure, communicate openly with your myoClinician. If the treatment feels overwhelming, let them know so they can adapt your treatment to your comfort level. The mind, body, and emotions are all connected, and shifts toward healing can be intense. When you feel emotional, treatment can be kept to a minimum. Discuss any concerns with your myoClinician to ensure a safe environment and an effective treatment experience.

Example: myoClinic Brentwood Bay

Let's use the myoClinic Brentwood Bay as an example. After completing the first three weekly appointments, follow-up sessions may be booked monthly, if needed. During the first three treatments, patients must pause intense workouts and activities to avoid full engagement or muscle strain after release to allow the body to recover and reset. Fully engaging muscles or pushing them to their limits after treatment can re-trigger tension and require repeating the treatment.

When monthly follow-up treatments start, the first week is for post-treatment recovery. In the second week, try gentle, short "testers" of activities (fifteen to twenty minutes, non-competitive), such as longer walks, hiking, kayaking, or golfing. If your body feels good, gradually increase time, effort, or weights used by about 10 percent each time—this can help rebuild your stamina without re-injury.

Remember, "start low, and go slow," and check in with the body often. Stretching after each activity helps lengthen muscles during recovery and helps prevent tightness. Also, avoid long periods of sitting (for instance, in the car) immediately after exercise to prevent stiffness and soreness.

"I can't tell you how much you're improving my life."

—myoActivation patient at the myoClinic Brentwood Bay, referred for persistent neck pain after a serious whiplash injury and severe restriction in movement

Chapter 9: What if it doesn't immediately feel better?

"As of late, we've been working on a shoulder injury and it's starting to return to a normal range of motion. If you want results, you have to be a willing participant on your healing journey. I'm so grateful we have this clinic on the South Island."

—Google review for the myoClinic Brentwood Bay

Key points

- You'll probably need multiple appointments to address your pain because chronic pain usually has multiple sources.
- You might experience a flare-up where your symptoms feel worse. If this happens, you can slow your treatment to avoid further flare-ups.
- If your muscles cramp, tell your clinician; this indicates that the area needs more treatment to release fully.
- Pain moving to other areas of the body is a good sign. It means that with continued treatment, you will start to feel better.
- If the pain returns, keep track of your activities between appointments to help identify any triggers.
- myoActivation can trigger the vagus nerve, sometimes causing nausea or light-headedness for a while after treatment. If you are prone to fainting after needles, arrange for someone to drive you home.

58

- If there is no improvement after several treatments, it is possible that the pain has a different source. In that case, discuss this with the doctor who referred you.
- Patience, open communication with your clinician, and following aftercare instructions closely will support faster healing.

Addressing chronic pain problems often requires several myoActivation sessions to work through various sources of myofascial dysfunction. Here are a few reasons why symptoms could feel worse initially:

Flare-ups

Some patients, especially those with widespread chronic pain, may experience flare-ups, where the body may feel sore, achy, and tired for three to five days, sometimes longer.

During flare-ups, staying hydrated, rest, and frequently changing postures throughout the day is crucial. Gentle walks and avoiding overexertion can also help. Open communication with your myoClinician can lead to tailored treatment that reduces flare-up frequency and duration. As body tension decreases with released areas, pain and fatigue also diminish, allowing for easier movement.

Cramping

Muscle cramping after needling suggests a partial release, which means that a portion of the muscle remains unable to relax fully. To release properly, the muscle may need more treatment. Contact your clinician if this occurs to ensure complete release and address the discomfort.

Shifting pain

As tension or discomfort resolves in one area, other tight or stressed areas may become more noticeable, sometimes even in distant body parts. This shifting sensation is considered a positive sign, reflecting the interconnected nature of the body. As layers of past injuries are resolved, like peeling an onion, you will start to notice the next layer.

Your myoClinician will focus on addressing the pain that is currently most intense. Therefore, changes in symptoms are seen as progress. Typically, discomfort in each subsequent area tends to be slightly less intense, indicating a gradual release of tension as treatment progresses.

Returning pain

If relief is initially short-lived, it is still a positive sign. With subsequent treatments of the dysfunctional areas, relief typically lasts longer. If pain returns, take a moment to reflect on the postures and activities performed in the past twenty-four hours that might have re-triggered strain. A pain journal (see Chapter 10) can help identify aggravating factors, for instance, track if extended periods of sitting or repetitive tasks are involved. Changing habits like alternating arms when vacuuming or getting up for a little stretch during ad breaks when watching a show can help prevent returning pain.

Non-pain symptoms

Some non-pain symptoms may include feeling woozy, changes in bowel habits, and tiredness. Shifts in body tension, especially around the abdomen, can stimulate the vagus nerve, which regulates the body's "rest and digest" functions. Vagus nerve stimulation can lead to symptoms like:

- brief nausea
- vomiting (very seldom)
- headache
- flushing or sweating
- fatigue
- dizziness or light-headedness
- lowered blood pressure (temporarily)

60

In some rare cases, syncope (fainting) may occur, especially in patients with a history of fainting after needles, for instance after blood tests or immunizations. It is recommended to bring someone to drive you home if you are prone to this.

No change

If there is no improvement after three or four sessions, it may be time to review possible non-myofascial underlying causes of pain. For instance, no response to myoActivation therapy may also signal that other stressful factors in life are creating a fight-or-flight reaction, tightening the body and changing the brain's perception of pain.

If chronic pain stems from an issue like a herniated disc compressing a nerve root, releasing muscle tension may only bring short-term relief as the root problem continues to create tension. Typically, most patients notice improvement within the first three treatments. However, if no improvement is observed, it is essential to acknowledge this fact honestly and reassess the treatment approach. It is always preferable to explore less invasive methods like myoActivation before considering stronger medications or more invasive procedures, which carry a higher risk of complications.

"I'm quite blown away actually."

—myoActivation patient treated for low back pain and stiffness

Chapter 10: What should I do after treatment?

"That's probably the easiest I've ever opened my jaw in my entire life."

—myoActivation patient

Key points

- Even as you start to feel better, continue following the aftercare instructions to maintain the benefits of the treatment.
- You may feel some shifting aches in different areas as your fascial system adjusts and realigns.
- Leading a healthy lifestyle and avoiding too much muscle strain will help you continue to feel better.

After treatment, even if you feel this wonderful sense of release, it is important to follow the aftercare instructions. This will help maintain the benefits of myoActivation treatment.

It is helpful to be mindful of the body's response after needling. The body adapts to these challenges when muscles, soft tissues, or scars have been under tension for an extended period. Releasing this tension can cause achiness in various areas as the fascial tissues realign and redistribute tension. Although this is a positive sign, the sensation may not feel pleasant due to the abundance of sensory nerves in the fascia that sense a change.[48]

62

Daily habits have a significant impact on overall well-being. If certain habits consistently create tension, strain muscles, or increase inflammation, the improvements from myoActivation treatment may not last. Therefore, prioritizing healthy habits and paying attention to the body's signals are crucial for maintaining a better quality of life.

Movement and posture

Key points

- Expect some achiness after treatment and take things easy until this subsides.
- Gentle, regular movement supports recovery, but avoid pushing yourself.
- Avoid staying in the same position for a long time. If driving or working at a desk, take breaks to stretch whenever possible.
- After the treatment, start with around a third of your usual exercise. If you don't feel stiff or sore the next day, you can slowly increase it as you continue to feel better.
- Gently stretch after exercising to prevent muscles from getting tight again.
- Listen to your body's signals—if it hurts, rest and try again later.
- Slow, steady progress will help keep the pain away.

During the first day or two after treatment, it's essential to rest and allow your body to adjust to the muscles being able to engage and release again. Avoid activities that push muscles to fatigue during this time. Gentle, regular movement helps keep your body warm and flexible, which supports recovery and helps the body adapt to changes in tension.

Each patient is unique, so proceed carefully if you feel any lingering achiness after treatment. Monitor your activity levels and the time you spend in postures. When ready to resume activities, start with around

30 percent of your usual activity level. For example, if you were used to walking for an hour each day before myoActivation, begin with a twenty-minute "test" walk after the treatment discomfort has eased. Muscles that were previously tight need to be strengthened gradually without strain.

The day after physical activity, check for any signs of stiffness or soreness. If present, they indicate that the muscles were overworked too soon and need more time to recover. Next time, reduce the activity duration or intensity and assess your body's reaction. If no soreness appears the following day, gradually increase the duration or intensity by about 10 percent at a time.

During the first week after treatment, the goal is gentle movement to prevent stiffness without straining the body. Immediately after treatment, avoid intense workouts or heavy lifting, as this is the period for muscles to reset and for tension to reorganize.

When treatment sensations have settled, slowly increase activity while being mindful of how your body feels. Stop if pain arises, assess what is happening, and consider adjusting posture or breaking up the tasks to support recovery.

Remember that muscles that have been tight or contracted for extended periods have lost strength because they have not been functioning fully. Once released, they can engage again, but it is easy to strain them. Patients often feel relieved of pain or stronger post-treatment and may be eager to resume various activities or chores previously avoided due to pain and dysfunction. However, overdoing it can quickly make the muscles strained, tight, and painful again.

Those who enjoy intense workouts (like weight training, high-intensity interval training, running, spinning, or cycling) may be familiar with the feeling of "good" stiffness and soreness the day after, which indicates to them an effective training session. However, as growth hormone levels decline with age (especially after the age of thirty-five),[49] the body heals less efficiently than in youth. Repeated intense workouts can increase muscle stiffness and fascia thickening, leading to reduced flexibility and mobility.

If you feel better even briefly after the treatment, this is a good sign that suggests a myofascial component to your symptoms. Gradually increasing activity is optimal, but this isn't always possible for everyone. If you must hold seated postures for prolonged periods (for work for example), the "sitting-time test" can help assess tolerance.

Sitting-time test

This test helps identify how long you can sit before feeling stiffness. Start by setting a twenty-minute timer while seated, then get up and assess how your body feels. If you don't experience any stiffness, increase the time by ten-minute increments, setting the timer for thirty minutes, then forty and so on. Some people notice stiffness quite quickly—even within ten minutes—while others can sit for up to 1.5 hours without issue. Knowing your own cut-off time for being seated allows you to stand and change posture before stiffness sets in, helping your body heal.

If you tend to focus deeply on tasks, set a timer to help remind you to get up, and/or to consider using a sit-stand desk to allow regular posture changes throughout the day.

Managing prolonged sitting

Driving can also lead to stiffness. If your "time to stiffness" is reached, break up your journey into smaller sections by stopping safely to walk for a minute or two and doing some gentle stretches.

Similarly, sitting in that comfortable corner of the couch every evening watching a favourite show can create stiffness. It is essential to change posture frequently enough to keep the body supple.

Like with driving, for physically demanding tasks such as building a deck or moving a house, pace yourself to prevent ending up in pain. This is especially important when engaging in activities that are not part of your daily routine. Changing postures and using different muscle groups every fifteen to twenty minutes or pacing the activity can ease the strain. Listen to your body and take brief breaks to prioritize your health over completing your to-do list quickly.

Avoiding prolonged sitting is best

Prolonged seated postures need to be avoided.[50] Regularly change posture when seated, especially during times of relaxation. When relaxing, people tend to sit in what feels like a comfortable position, which may not be ideal and, over time, cause asymmetrical changes in tissues. These changes may result in stiffening and shortening of the muscle, which in turn makes it harder for the body to move freely afterward. Alternating seating positions, getting up and standing, walking around, or stretching every twenty to thirty minutes can keep your body supple.

Finding sources of stiffness or discomfort

If you notice stiffness or achiness, consider what activities or postures may have triggered it. It may be something about your habits, behaviour, or environment, and changes must be made to prevent symptoms.

Reviewing activities in the previous twenty-four hours can reveal prolonged postures (like sitting), repetitive movements, or activities that may have been less than ideal ergonomically. If discomfort increases after sleep, assess your mattress and sleep position as potential sources of the issue. For instance, consider whether the mattress requires replacement; you may also experiment with various sleeping postures, supports, and strategies to identify what can alleviate the discomfort. Additional suggestions include trying a memory foam mattress topper or using small supports, like a pillow, under your waist and between the knees (especially for side sleepers) to improve comfort.

Post-activity stretching

As you start feeling better and resume activities gently, incorporate gentle stretching after hiking, biking, or pickleball for example to release muscle tension. Stretching after the workout needs to be as much a priority as the workout itself, especially if you've dealt with myofascial strain in the past.

Gentle stretching is also beneficial at other times, such as after prolonged periods of sitting, for example, when driving. Consider breaking up any drive longer than thirty minutes by stopping somewhere safe and walking around the car for a minute to let things stretch and loosen up.

Hydration, nutrition, and supplementation

Key points

- Drinking water is essential for managing chronic pain, supporting faster healing and reducing stress.
- A balanced diet with unprocessed foods, vegetables, and lean proteins can help you recover from pain.
- Specific supplements can also help during recovery, but you should also consult your doctor or a dietician for guidance.

Hydration

Good hydration is crucial after procedures like myoActivation, especially in the context of chronic pain management, offering benefits like:

- **Facilitating healing:** Proper hydration supports the body's natural healing processes, especially important after needling.

After trigger point injections, the body responds to the micro-injuries from the needle with bruising and mild inflammation to heal. Proper hydration supports tissue repair and clears waste products, promoting recovery.[51]

- **Minimizing side effects and enhancing detoxification:** Some patients may experience mild side effects after needling, such as swelling or tenderness. This happens because long-contracted tissues release built-up metabolic waste, sometimes causing a feeling of fatigue.[52] Proper hydration supports the body's natural detoxification processes by helping to flush out toxins and metabolic waste.

- **Maintaining electrolyte balance:** Hydration supports electrolyte balance in the body, which is essential for proper nerve function, muscle contractions, and overall physiological stability. Sometimes, when you have been sweating heavily (for instance, due to heat or intense training), low-sugar electrolyte drinks (like Hydralyte) can help restore balance.[53]

- **Promoting general well-being:** Chronic pain increases physical and emotional stress and tension.[54] Dehydration can worsen stress and contribute to fatigue and irritability, while hydration can help ease these feelings.

Dehydration

Dehydration can show up in weight changes, dry mouth, thirst, or reduced skin elasticity (for instance, when hydrated, if you pinch the skin on the back of the hand, it should bounce back), urine output and colour. Dehydration can also be confirmed in the clinical setting by blood tests. Check the urine colour at home: Good hydration is associated with pale straw-coloured urine, while darker, amber or light brown urine indicates dehydration.[55] In chronic pain management, hydration is essential not only after myoActivation procedures but also as part of an ongoing self-care routine.

Nutrition

For people living with chronic pain, maintaining a healthy diet can be challenging. Comfort eating, limited energy for meal prep, or turning to easy take-out can lead to nutrient imbalances and may increase pain and inflammation.[56] [57]

Nutrition matters, and good nutrition can help in managing chronic pain and support overall well-being.[58] For instance, a balanced diet can help reduce inflammation, promote tissue repair, and provide essential support for the body's natural healing processes. To achieve and maintain a balanced diet and support your body, consider the following tips:

- **Emphasize fruits and vegetables:** Rich in antioxidants, vitamins, and nutrients, fruits and vegetables help combat inflammation. Make multiple portions when you cook and freeze extra meals for those days when you feel overwhelmed or are just not up for cooking.
- **Choose healthy fats:** Alongside omega-3 fatty acids, incorporate healthy fats from sources like olive oil, avocados, and nuts, which have anti-inflammatory benefits.
- **Include lean protein:** High-quality protein sources like tofu, legumes, fish, lean meats, and poultry provide essential amino acids for tissue repair and overall health. It has been shown that plant-based protein has less inflammatory properties than animal-based protein.[59]
- **Limit processed foods:** Processed foods are often high in sugars, unhealthy fats, preservatives, stabilizers, and chemicals, which can worsen inflammation. When ordering take-out, opt for poke bowls, pho, or other options that contain whole foods and are not deep fried.

Supplements

Additionally, certain supplements, such as omega-3 fatty acids, magnesium bis-glycinate, vitamin K2, vitamin B12[60] and vitamin D3, can support chronic pain management.

When considering supplements, it's essential to consult a healthcare provider or a registered dietitian to find appropriate dosages and avoid interactions with any medications or medical conditions for a particular individual. Supplements should complement a well-balanced diet, not replace it. Rich in various nutrients, whole foods provide additional benefits beyond isolated or synthetic supplements.

Omega-3 fatty acids

Omega-3 fatty acids have anti-inflammatory properties that can help reduce inflammation associated with chronic and inflammatory pain conditions like rheumatoid arthritis and osteoarthritis.[61]

Sources of omega-3 fatty acids include fatty fish (salmon, mackerel, anchovies, and sardines). Vegan omega-3 fatty acids supplements are sourced from flaxseed, chia seeds and walnuts.

Vitamin K2

Vitamin K2 is essential for bone health as it helps regulate calcium metabolism,[62] directing it to bones and clearing it from tendons and arteries. Maintaining strong bones can be particularly important for individuals with chronic pain conditions like osteoporosis or back pain.

Vitamin K2 is found in fermented foods, certain cheeses, and in smaller amounts in meat and eggs, and K2 supplements can be taken if dietary intake is low.

Vitamin D3

Vitamin D3 is vital for overall bone health, immune support, and reducing inflammation. It also helps the body absorb calcium and maintain proper bone density.[63] Vitamin D3 may be particularly helpful for individuals with chronic pain conditions, especially those with musculoskeletal pain or fibromyalgia who may have lower vitamin D levels.

Vitamin D3 can be obtained from sunlight exposure and dietary sources such as fatty fish, fortified dairy products, and egg yolks. Supplements may be necessary for those with inadequate sun exposure or specific medical conditions.

Finding balance

Key points

- Chronic pain is exhausting, and so is healing. Be patient with yourself and listen to your body's needs.
- Finding balance and pacing yourself can help keep the pain away.
- Take breaks from long periods of sitting or physical work and stretch regularly. After muscles are released, they need time to regain strength.
- Take care of your mental health, as it affects physical pain. Lean on loved ones and consider getting help from a therapist or doctor if needed.
- Meditation and stretching can reduce stress.
- Spend time with those you care about; loneliness can worsen your health.
- Prioritise time for yourself, and if you need workplace accommodations (like a sit-to-stand desk or a flexible schedule), ask for them. Your clinician can provide support documentation.

- Ensure quality sleep—a cool, dark room and a consistent bedtime routine can improve your rest.
- Drink plenty of water and eat fresh, unprocessed foods.
- Consult a physiotherapist to support your recovery.

Achieving balance is crucial for coping with chronic pain and improving overall well-being and quality of life. Chronic pain is often both physically and emotionally draining and pacing yourself is vital to prevent setbacks. Valuable self-management resources are available at www.liveplanbe.ca for adults and mycarepath.ca for youth.

It's common for those with "type A" personalities—those who push themselves emotionally, physically, and generally in life—to experience pain syndromes. So, it's no coincidence that a substantial proportion of the patients who get referred for pain treatment have "type A" personalities.[64] Recovery often involves learning to listen to the body and balance physical and emotional demands. Once tension is released and pain is reduced through myoActivation, it's essential to regain stamina gradually, carefully, and without strain. To prevent setbacks, it is also important to heed any discomfort and avoid "pushing through" it.

Physical activity

Pacing daily activities and interspersing periods of rest can help manage pain levels. Overexertion and excessive physical activity may exacerbate pain, and being too sedentary can lead to muscle stiffness and deconditioning. After myoActivation, soft tissues have been released, but muscles may be weakened due to not functioning normally, especially if the pain has been present for a long time.

Emotional health

Chronic pain can significantly impact emotional well-being, often causing stress, anxiety, and depression,[65] which in turn can also cause more pain.

Finding emotional balance involves recognizing, accepting, and expressing feelings, seeking support from loved ones or a therapist, and practicing mindfulness and relaxation techniques. This is important because emotional balance can help break the cycle of pain and tension.

For instance, anxiety and stress can exacerbate bodily tension, creating a cycle of discomfort which activates the fight-and-flight system (sympathetic nervous system) of the body. Breathing techniques and stretching, which activate the parasympathetic nervous system (the "rest-and-digest" system), can help alleviate tension, anxiety, and stress. Furthermore, mindfulness practices, meditation,[66] and hypnosis[67] can help individuals manage pain and reduce stress.[68] Taking time for self-care activities, such as gentle exercise, relaxation techniques, hobbies, and spending time in nature, can help individuals recharge and manage stress related to chronic pain. Additionally, taking brief breaks during stressful days to organize thoughts and break down large tasks into smaller, more manageable steps is helpful.[69]

Visit www.bcalm.ca for more useful techniques on managing emotional balance.

Social connections

Chronic pain can sometimes lead to social isolation, as individuals may withdraw from social activities. Maintaining a balance in social connections is vital for emotional support and reducing feelings of loneliness and isolation.[70]

Work-life balance

Balancing work responsibilities with personal life can help manage chronic pain. Taking breaks, pacing activities, and requesting workplace accommodations, such as a sit-to-stand desk, can help maintain physical health while supporting productivity. If needed, myoClinicians can provide documentation to support workplace accommodation requests.

At work and home, it is important to avoid extended periods of sitting in front of a screen (TV, computer, cell phone), and change postures regularly to maintain a healthy body and reduce pain.

Sleep

Good sleep supports pain management and overall health. Creating a sleep-friendly environment by establishing a consistent bedtime routine in a fully dark and cool environment can improve sleep quality and reduce pain-related sleep issues.

Nutrition

A balanced, nutrient-rich diet can support overall health and well-being. Proper nutrition can reduce inflammation and increase energy levels, which can affect how you perceive pain. Limiting processed and high-sugar foods and drinks (including pop and alcohol) can lessen inflammation and improve energy levels.

Physical therapy

Working with a professional who can design a personalized exercise plan after myoActivation treatment can help build stamina, supporting long-term recovery.

Working with professionals

Finding balance in physical activity, emotional health, social connections, and nutrition can significantly improve the quality of life for those living with chronic pain. A team of healthcare professionals—including pain specialists, physical therapists, and counsellors—especially if there is a history of trauma, can create a comprehensive pain management plan that supports balance and well-being across all spheres of life.

Pain journaling

Key points

- If you have trouble tracking your pain, try keeping a pain journal.
- A pain journal records what you were doing and how you felt, helping you follow your recovery and identify anything that makes the pain worse.
- In the pain journal, write down the date, what you were doing, where you felt pain, and what the pain felt like.
- A blank pain journal template, pain scale, and prompts for describing pain are available in this chapter.
- Check in with your body when you notice you're in pain, but don't dwell on it—focusing too much on pain can make it feel worse.
- Sharing your pain journal with your doctor or clinician can help them treat you effectively.

Starting a pain journal

Keeping a journal can be helpful for patients who struggle to remember their pain experiences, how activities affected them, or fluctuations in symptoms. Pain often shifts, making it hard to recollect details over time. Once treatment starts, a journal can help track and recall experiences and capture pain changes, especially when pain diminishes or vanishes. But it's important to avoid focusing too much on pain because attention can amplify it.

Maintaining a journal helps identify patterns, triggers, and any improvements in pain management to guide your treatment. Below is a simple journal template:

Pain journal template

- **Date:** Write down the date.
- **Pain score:** Use a scale from 0 to 10 to rate your pain, with 0 as no pain and 10 as the worst pain imaginable. Note the area that feels the worst when tracking changes.

Pain score guidelines

- 0: No pain
- 1–3: Mild pain (tolerable, doesn't interfere with daily activities)
- 4–6: Moderate pain (noticeable, may affect daily activities)
- 7–8: Severe pain (strong, limits daily activities)
- 9–10: Excruciating pain (unbearable)

If multiple areas are involved, add additional information to help identify triggers:

- **Pain description:** Describe the type of pain with one word, such as sharp, dull, throbbing, or burning.
- **Location:** Indicate where the pain is localized, using a body diagram, if helpful. If you have multiple areas, pick the three most prominent and rate each.
- **Activities:** Note the activities you were involved in during the twenty-four hours before pain changed or increased, for instance, sitting, walking, exercising, or working at a desk.
- **Triggers:** Identify any possible pain triggers, such as physical activity, prolonged postures, stress, or weather changes.
- **Sleep quality:** Include a brief note about how you slept the previous night.

- **Mood/Emotions:** Write down your emotional state/how stressed you are for the day, as stress and emotions (such as anxiety states) can affect pain perception and cause increased muscular tension.[71]

Tips for keeping the pain journal

- **Be consistent:** Record your pain levels and other details whenever you notice a change or become aware of pain triggers.
- **Take notes:** Jot down any additional observations, changes in pain patterns, or questions you may have for your healthcare provider.
- **Share with healthcare providers:** Your pain journal can provide helpful information for your myoClinician.
- **Use technology:** Consider using digital diaries or calendars for easier and more accessible tracking.

Remember that a pain journal is a tool for tracking, not for focusing on pain. It should be adapted to meet your needs and preferences. With time, identifying patterns and gaining insights can support more effective management of pain and better communication with your healthcare team.

Monday	Tuesday	Wednes.	Thursday	Friday	Saturday	Sunday
Date:	Date:	Date:	Date:	Date:	Date:	Date:
Pain location and type:	Pain location and type:	Pain location and type:	Pain location and type:	Pain location and type:	Pain location and type:	Pain location and type:
Pain score:	Pain score:	Pain score:	Pain score:	Pain score:	Pain score:	Pain score:
Date:	Date:	Date:	Date:	Date:	Date:	Date:
Pain location and type:	Pain location and type:	Pain location and type:	Pain location and type:	Pain location and type:	Pain location and type:	Pain location and type:
Pain score:	Pain score:	Pain score:	Pain score:	core:	Pain score:	Pain score:
Date:	Date:	Date:	Date:	Date:	Date:	Date:
Pain location and type:	Pain location and type:	Pain location and type:	Pain location and type:	Pain location and type:	Pain location and type:	Pain location and type:
Pain score:	Pain score:	Pain score:	Pain score:	Pain score:	Pain score:	Pain score:
Date:	Date:	Date:	Date:	Date:	Date:	Date:
Pain location and type:	Pain location and type:	Pain location and type:	Pain location and type:	Pain location and type:	Pain location and type:	Pain location and type:
Pain score:	Pain score:	Pain score:	Pain score:	Pain score:	Pain score:	Pain score:

Chapter 11: Special considerations for myoActivation

"It took a year of treatments, but I have virtually eliminated migraines after suffering for over sixty years! Give it a try; nothing to lose, except your headaches!
Check out myoActivation on Google and read the science behind it."
—Google review for the myoClinic Brentwood Bay

myoActivation is designed to provide relief from chronic pain by releasing tension in the muscles and fascia. However, certain groups of people may have additional considerations or need tailored approaches due to specific health circumstances or unique challenges. This chapter explores considerations and guidelines for different individuals seeking myoActivation, whether they are pregnant, over sixty-five, living with cognitive impairments, transitioning, or dealing with trauma-related pain.

myoActivation considerations during pregnancy

Key points

- Any medical treatment during pregnancy can impact the developing fetus; however, untreated pain or stress can also be harmful.
- During the first trimester, it's best to avoid any myoActivation treatment unless your pain is too much to manage.
- After the first trimester, light treatment away from the abdomen and uterus may provide relief.
- Since myoActivation contains no chemicals or drugs, it is safer than many other pain treatments during pregnancy.

Pregnant patients who are familiar with myoActivation often request treatment for painful symptoms like migraines or lower back pain. During pregnancy, the body's hormones constantly change, and medical care providers typically aim to keep interventions to a minimum during pregnancy; however, stress hormones released in response to pain can also affect the fetus and its environment.[72]

If pain relief is necessary, myoActivation can be utilized cautiously, avoiding the lower abdomen or uterus area. Pregnant patients often appreciate the relief and the reduced need for medication. However, each case is individually assessed. Because pregnancy is most vulnerable during the first trimester, treatment is avoided during this time unless the patient's pain severity and debilitation outweigh other risks.

myoActivation, free from any drugs or chemicals that can affect the development of the fetus, is generally a safer option than most medication-based pain treatments during pregnancy.

myoActivation can help with widespread chronic pain

Key points

- For those with central sensitivity syndrome or other widespread chronic pain like fibromyalgia, part of the problem could be coming from the body (tight muscles and fascia) and part from the brain.
- myoActivation can help pain management and improve mobilty.

Widespread chronic pain conditions, such as fibromyalgia and central sensitization syndromes, can cause widespread body pain, stiffness, weakness, muscle fatigue, and chronic generalized fatigue.[73] This pain is often described as fluctuating, and even light touch can feel painful. The reasons for this increased sensitivity to pain are not fully understood, but changes in the central nervous system and the muscles and soft tissues likely contribute.

One theory suggests that certain chemicals in the body make the nerves more sensitive to pain signals, whether those signals come from the true source of pain (for instance, muscle pressure) or something typically non-painful (like a light touch). Another theory suggests that the brain becomes sensitized to pain signals, amplifying the pain perception (a process called centralization). It's possible that myofascial dysfunction in the core soft tissues of the body can distort nerve signals in the fascial system and heighten pain sensitivity. When fascial injuries are linked with traumatic events, they may also stimulate the brain's pain centres.

Although science has yet to understand these chronic pain conditions fully, evidence suggests that both heightened nerve sensitivity in the brain and changes in local tissues contribute to pain. myoActivation can help relieve the pain burden by treating localized conditions. Patients treated with myoActivation often report improved mobility, reduced pain and tension, better sleep and improved overall well-being.

myoActivation in later life stages

Key points

- Many older adults experience chronic pain and may be sensitive to medications, making access to pain relief difficult.
- myoActivation can relieve pain without adding more medications, supporting a better quality of life and greater independence.

Chronic pain is common in older adults, who are often more sensitive to medication. They may experience increased side effects, such as balance issues or risk of falls. In addition, older adults may face financial constraints, social isolation, depression, or difficulty performing daily tasks, all of which can challenge their independence. Chronic pain can also impact their quality of life considerably.

Pharmacological approaches to chronic pain management in adults in later life often can provide only limited relief and can cause side effects, such as urinary retention, constipation, sedation, cognitive decline, and a higher risk of falls. Unfortunately, older individuals are often underrepresented in clinical trials for chronic pain treatments, leaving uncertainties about the effects of multiple medications taken simultaneously and physical frailty, on treatment outcomes and side effects. Balancing expected pain relief with potential risks of side effects presents an ongoing challenge.[74]

Persistent pain has been associated with a faster cognitive decline and a higher risk of developing dementia. Research shows that persistent pain may lead to more severe depressive symptoms, limits in daily activities, faster memory decline, and increased difficulty maintaining independence, both financially and in life in general.[75]

Reducing persistent pain can significantly improve the quality of life and preserve independence for adults in later life. myoActivation reduces pain without adding to the pharmacological burden or causing interactions with other medications patients take. Finally, it can be a cost-effective option within healthcare systems and for individuals.

myoActivation for patients with dementia or cognitive impairment

Key points

- People with dementia or cognitive impairment may struggle to communicate their pain, leading to undertreated symptoms.
- Family members or caregivers may not know how much pain the person with dementia or cognitive impairment is experiencing.
- myoActivation offers a quick, affordable, non-medicated option for pain relief.
- If a person with dementia or cognitive impairment cannot consent to treatment, a caregiver or legal representative may need to do so on their behalf.

Chronic pain is common among individuals with dementia and cognitive impairment, significantly affecting their overall well-being and quality of life. As cognitive function declines, it can be harder for individuals to communicate their pain effectively, leading to underestimation or mismanagement of pain symptoms.

This makes obtaining informed consent for medical treatments challenging since dementia and cognitive impairment can hinder the ability to understand treatment options, as well as their potential risks and benefits. A legal guardian or person with medical power of attorney (a substitute decision-maker or healthcare representative) may need to consent to treatment on their behalf, if the individual cannot do so.

Untreated or inadequately managed pain may worsen behavioural symptoms associated with dementia, such as agitation and aggression, affecting the individual's ability to perform daily activities and interact with others. Addressing chronic pain in people with dementia and cognitive impairment can significantly improve their quality of life by reducing discomfort, enhancing functional abilities, and potentially reducing the need for additional supports, sedative or psychotropic medications.

myoActivation is especially suitable for this population, as it involves no additional chemicals, provides quick relief, is cost-effective and helps preserve independence.

myoActivation in palliative care

Key points

- If you're in palliative care, myoActivation can help make you more comfortable.
- Even if another condition means you can't take ordinary pain medication, myoActivation can help control your pain.
- Pain relief during end-of-life care is essential for comfort and dignity, benefiting the patient and their caregivers.

Pain control is critically important in palliative and end-of-life care to ease discomfort and support the patient's sense of dignity. At this sensitive stage, managing pain effectively ensures that patients can experience peace and comfort, alleviating the emotional strain on those involved in their care.

Pain relief in palliative and end-of-life care can be challenging due to the complexity of pain syndromes combined with multiple concurrent symptoms and the patient's physical decline. Despite these challenges, prioritizing pain control in end-of-life care remains crucial to helping patients find comfort and peace.

myoActivation is especially well-suited for palliative care as it is simple, drug-free, provides quick relief, and requires no specialized equipment. This approach to pain management supports comfort, is gentle on the body, and can be seamlessly integrated into a palliative care plan.

myoActivation after gender reassignment

Key points

- Transgender people are more likely to experience chronic pain due to factors like stress, gender dysphoria, and surgical scarring.
- Scarring from top or bottom surgeries can cause chronic pain and limit movement.
- Transgender people may have trouble accessing appropriate healthcare, which may make managing pain more difficult.
- myoActivation can help reduce pain, improve mobility, and support overall well-being during the transition process.

Research shows that transgender individuals may experience higher rates of chronic pain compared to the general population.[76] Contributing factors include the physical and emotional stress associated with gender dysphoria, hormone therapy, and surgical interventions.

Gender-affirming surgeries, such as chest reconstruction (top surgery) and genital reconstruction (bottom surgery), are often key steps in the transition journey. Still, they can create significant scarring that can affect movement and lead to chronic pain. For instance, chest surgery leaves scars along the chest wall, an area of the body that requires elasticity to facilitate breathing and shoulder movement. Restricted movement in these areas can contribute to ongoing discomfort.

Additionally, transgender individuals may also face challenges in accessing adequate pain management and support services, further worsening their pain experiences.

It is crucial to acknowledge and address the potential impact of chronic pain because it can contribute to the success of transitioning and improve the overall quality of life for transgender individuals. myoActivation can help alleviate pain from scar tissue, improve mobility, and reduce overall pain, supporting a smoother transition process.

myoActivation when hypermobile

Key points

- Hypermobility, where joints are unusually flexible, often causes chronic pain and discomfort.
- Careful treatment using myoActivation can help soothe the connective tissues, though treatment may need to proceed slowly.
- Targeted strengthening exercises can help prevent further strain or injury.

Hypermobility, a genetic condition characterized by joints moving beyond the normal ranges, often results in pain due to the added strain on connective tissues. This condition relates to specific types of collagen, which is the main protein that provides structure to connective tissues such as ligaments and tendons, and their functions within the body. People with hypermobility may have alterations in the collagen structure, which affect tissue stability and elasticity. There is a large spectrum of hypermobility syndromes, from what is considered benign to more severe presentations, such as Ehlers-Danlos syndrome.[77]

Fibroblasts, the cells responsible for producing collagen, play a crucial role in maintaining the integrity and stability of connective tissues. In individuals with hypermobility, fewer fibroblasts in connective tissues may lead to disruptions in collagen production and tissue stability, resulting in slower healing.

Excessive joint mobility can strain ligaments and tendons, causing inflammation and discomfort. Moreover, stretching beyond a safe range can jeopardize joint stability, making injuries such as sprains, strains, and dislocations more likely.

Joint hypermobility syndromes can also manifest with gastrointestinal symptoms, sleep disorders, fibromyalgia, psychological disorders, migraine headaches, ophthalmic issues, and nervous system dysfunction, among other associated conditions.[78]

There are a few indicators of hypermobility. For adults, the following questions have been used to screen for hypermobility:

- Can you now (or could you ever) place your hands flat on the floor without bending your knees?
- Can you now (or could you ever) bend your thumb to touch your forearm?
- As a child, did you amuse your friends by contorting your body into strange shapes or doing the splits?
- As a child or teenager, did your shoulder or kneecap dislocate on more than one occasion?
- Do you consider yourself double-jointed (which describes joints that can move beyond their normal range, allowing for positions most people cannot achieve)?

If the answer is "yes" to two or more of these questions, there is a strong likelihood that the person falls on the hypermobile spectrum.

myoActivation can help relieve discomfort in areas with sustained contraction and restore balance in posture. Treatment typically takes a cautious, minimalistic approach to avoid compromising joint stability.[79] Targeted exercises to strengthen supporting muscles while avoiding excessive joint extension can help reduce pain and minimize future injury.

"That feels so much nicer already."

—myoActivation patient

Chapter 12: myoActivation for kids or youth

by Dr Gillian Lauder

"I'm not sure I have ever felt this happy in six years. You know when the first warm sun after winter is over? That's what it feels like. It feels absolutely amazing."

—a twelve-year-old with long-standing chronic low back pain, at discharge after three myoActivation sessions

Key points

- If you're a kid or teenager with chronic pain, myofascial dysfunction could be a part of it.
- Scars from trauma, injury, and surgery can cause MFD in kids and teenagers. Doing hard, repetitive movements, having poor posture, or overusing your muscles can also contribute.
- Treatment for pain in kids and teenagers is often slow and careful, focusing on foundational approaches, illustrated in this section by a pyramid—starting from the bottom and moving upwards.
- myoActivation can help non-verbal kids and teenagers who may struggle to describe and communicate their pain.

- If you're scared of doctors or needles, that's okay—there are ways the clinician can help make it easier for you.
- myoActivation can also provide information to help your doctor understand and treat your pain.

Many young people have unrecognized myofascial dysfunction[80] as a component of their chronic pain.[81] This dysfunction can develop in response to trauma, injury, surgery, repetitive physical activities, poor posture, muscle overuse, or overload. Scars are common in the pediatric population and can contribute to pain even when they appear "normal."[82] An advantage of myoActivation is that it can easily identify myofascial components of pain in children and youth, although conservative approaches are usually recommended before proceeding to myoActivation.

For young people, returning to normal function is always the primary goal in chronic pain therapy. Managing chronic pain in young people can be visualized as a pyramid (see Figure 2), with conservative management as the base of the pyramid. Lifestyle education and adjustments—such as paced activities, good nutrition, and sleep hygiene—are typically the first steps.

An interdisciplinary approach, including physiotherapy (and massage), psychology, and pharmacology (the 3Ps), has proven effective in reducing pain, improving physical function and mood and supporting school attendance for young people living with chronic pain (see mycarepath.ca for more information).[83] The base of the pyramid is where the journey to recovery begins. Progressing up the steps of this pyramid of care addresses the various factors contributing to each young person's unique experience of chronic pain.

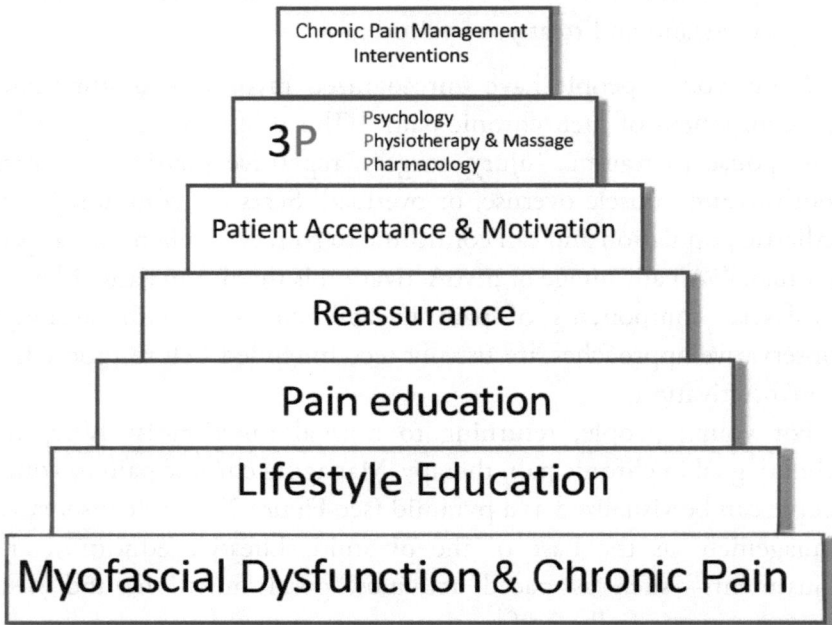

Figure 2 The pyramid of care.

A myofascial component of pain is diagnosed through myoActivation movement tests and examination for scars and areas of pain. When myofascial pain is identified, conservative measures, such as supplementation with magnesium, vitamin K2, and Vitamin D3 may be recommended to help relax tight muscles. Often, these steps lead to a noticeable improvement in tension.

When the myofascial component of pain persists, myoActivation may be considered, but this depends on the child's age and developmental stage. If deemed appropriate treatment, myoActivation is introduced as a therapy during the initial assessment and is supported with verbal and written information. myoActivation can be a useful tool in managing chronic pain related to myofascial dysfunction in young people and has been shown to improve pain and mobility.[84]

Using myoActivation in children and youth presents unique challenges. For those children and youth who have needle aversion (fear of needles) or have anxiety related to medical procedures, a careful risk-benefit analysis is done on an individual basis. Non-pharmacological techniques, including introducing distraction, modification of breathing techniques, music, virtual reality, or mobile devices, to reduce needle-related pain are always employed in pediatric patients.

Topical anesthetic cream (for example, EMLA) can be applied to the target areas (especially scars) about an hour before the appointment to minimize the discomfort. Vapocoolant spray (cold spray) is also another useful option. Sedative medications may be added when these methods aren't enough to manage the child's anxiety and needle pain. If needed, IV sedation with anesthetic monitoring can be used.

For younger or nonverbal children, assessment may be limited by their ability to cooperate or follow commands. In these cases, the clinician needs to rely on parental or guardian observations to identify problem areas, using experience to find muscles in sustained contraction or fascial tension. Sedation may be necessary for young and nonverbal children.

myoActivation is a valuable tool for diagnosing and treating chronic pain in young people, often revealing myofascial issues that otherwise go unnoticed. The relief that young people experience from myoActivaton is often profound, even after many years of pain and trying other therapies.

As one young patient described:

"There were several times in my treatments when I saw things I thought couldn't be changed and were just 'the way they were' change significantly because they were actually being caused by stored tension that could then be released. My posture has become visibly more symmetric, my surgical scars have diminished, and I've gained mobility I didn't even think was possible. Throughout the whole process, my pain steadily

decreased, and I could do more and more between each session, which allowed me to gain my strength back and recover much faster. I'm so grateful to have been able to receive myoActivation treatment."

Chapter 13: myoActivation and pain associated with trauma

by Barb Eddy

"I feel definitely more balanced."
—myoActivation patient

Key points

- When you experience an injury under stressful or traumatic conditions, your nervous system "remembers" it, even when you don't consciously recall it.
- Moving the injured area, even after it heals, can trigger these subconscious memories, causing symptoms like pain, anxiety, brain fog, nausea, fatigue, or headaches.
- Treating the myofascial tissue in the injured area can reduce these symptoms.
- During treatment, you might experience feelings or memories related to the trauma, even if you don't remember it consciously. If this becomes overwhelming, your clinician can adjust or pause treatment to help you cope.
- Processing these emotions can eventually lead to feelings of hope and relief.

myoActivation is designed to treat chronic pain and dysfunction, but it can also help relieve the suffering associated with traumatic injuries. Research is exploring how trauma can "embed" emotions and memories of events within the body's soft tissues, including the fascial system, and parts of the brain.[85] Fascia, a type of connective tissue with many nerves, links different layers of tissue from skin to bone throughout the body.

When fascia is injured—especially in stressful or traumatic situations—it undergoes changes in its structure, movement and function, which can also affect how it interacts with the brain's pain centers.[86] Chronic pain and trauma-related pain may share pathways in the nervous system,[87] [88] meaning that physical injury can connect with the memory and emotions to produce whole-body effects. The book *The Body Keeps the Score*, by psychiatrist Dr Bessel Van Der Kolk,[89] explains this link between emotions, memory, and the body well (please note that this book contains descriptions that may be difficult to read for those with trauma).

A common example of this nervous system connection is a person who has been in a serious car accident. They will likely have soft tissue damage over their chest along the line of the seatbelt, and the brain memory centres might imprint both the physical injury and stress associated with the accident together. Later, movements involving the chest area, like breathing, may bring up feelings of anxiety, even though the physical injury has healed.

Trauma-informed myoActivation

myoActivation can be highly effective when approached with a trauma-informed perspective that supports the person's emotional well-being and healing. While there are no formal studies available on this yet, myoClinicians have seen patients recall past events and experience strong emotions during treatment for injuries related to trauma, when traumatically injured soft tissues are needled. Reactions range from brief reflections to vivid memories, often accompanied by emotional release.

These responses to needling are often surprising to patients, who may need a moment to process the experience. The good news is that after an emotional needling experience, clinicians have also witnessed patients feeling hopeful, energized, and uplifted. Needling the injured myofascial tissues modifies how signals travel through the nervous system, "turning down" the intensity of the link between the injury and memory. As a result, patients may feel less anxiety, tension, and pain. Often, changes are positive in the way a person relates to their past experiences. Some patients report improved focus and sleep, while many feel a general sense of relief. Counselling can be helpful, and patients may also find they need fewer pain medications or other substances (including drugs and alcohol) for pain management.

Because everyone's emotional response to myoActivation is different, it is important to prepare for needling before the treatment. Both the clinician and patient benefit from a trauma-informed approach, and it can be helpful to discuss past injuries with the myoClinician before the treatment. Persons who have experienced physical, emotional, and sexual trauma may be particularly sensitive, but even physical scars from surgeries or childhood accidents can hold tension. Practicing relaxation techniques before and after the treatment can help, and if a strong emotional response is anticipated, the myoActivation session can be delayed while the patient prepares for the treatment and organizes post-care support. Those living with pain are often the best experts on their bodies, emotions, and history of injury.

A trauma-informed approach also places the person in the centre of the myoActivation process, tailoring the treatment to suit the individual and their pain. In addition to considering physical and emotional injuries and impaired mobility, it is also important to address the patient's current needs and responsibilities, such as work, home and social life.

Supporting the healing process

For the best myoActivation results, consider activities that calm the nervous system, such as outdoor time, yoga, lighthearted TV shows, and reducing time spent on social media. A calmer nervous system can have lasting effects on physical, emotional, and social well-being. myoActivation can play a unique role in holistic healing from chronic pain, especially for those carrying pain linked to trauma.

> *"Oh wow! That's crazy. It's completely different.*
> *That's insane. Huge difference!"*

—a patient after receiving myoActivation treatment

Chapter 14: Conclusion

*"I find that feeling the changes in the body with treatment
is emotional, but they are happy tears. I would like to
continue treatment as much as possible despite the tears. I'm
experiencing waves of stuff at the end of the appointment."*

—myoActivation patient, after treating severe
burn scars from their childhood

Key points

- One in five adults has experienced chronic pain at some point.
- Pain treatment is often ineffective, complicated, expensive, or difficult to access.
- myoActivation offers a simple, low-cost, and effective solution.
- The process starts with reviewing your medical history, followed by assessing posture and movement tests.
- During the treatment, thin needles are inserted into tight muscles, scars, or distorted fascial tissue to facilitate release. The needles are immediately removed after insertion.

- The body's healing response kicks in after treatment, soothing and loosening the muscles, tissues, or scars. This promotes improved movement and reduces pain.
- myoActivation can reduce chronic pain and make daily life easier.

One in five adults have a lived experience of chronic pain[90]. Thanks to the work of Dr. Gregory Siren, a groundbreaking approach to assessing and treating myofascial components of chronic pain is available through myoActivation. This treatment has the potential to revolutionize chronic pain care, offering an effective, accessible, and low-cost solution in a field where such options are often limited.

One of the unique aspects of myoActivation is its detailed approach to assessment. Unlike conventional medical history-taking, myoActivation begins with a detailed review of a patient's lifetime trauma timeline, including surgeries, injuries, and even seemingly minor elements like chickenpox scars. Postural assessment and movement assessments further help identify specific areas that need treatment, providing a comprehensive view of the body's dysfunction.

Treatment involves inserting fine needles into tight muscles, scars, or distorted fascia. This process stimulates a controlled healing response in the body, leading to pain reduction, improved flexibility, enhanced range of motion, and improved overall well-being. Unlike some needling techniques, myoActivation uses fine-gauge hypodermic needles and a minimally invasive approach, providing relief without leaving needles in the body or adding stimuli like electricity. Treatments and assessments occur in cycles, allowing the clinician to identify and address different dysfunctional areas over time.

myoActivation can help with a wide range of pain conditions, from general back pain to arthritis-related discomfort, pain and tenderness in the jaw joints and surrounding muscles, and even scar-related pain. By targeting specific tissues—scars, muscles, and fascia—myoActivation triggers a healing response, improves blood flow, and reduces tension, offering relief for many chronic pain issues.

The benefits of myoActivation go beyond pain relief. Patients report improved functionality, range of motion, independence, and emotional release from past trauma stored in the body. For those seeking lasting relief and a better quality of life, myoActivation provides a hopeful and effective approach.

"I am feeling fantastic!"

—myoActivation patient

Contributing Authors

Barb Eddy BSN, MN, NP(F)

Barb Eddy is a nurse practitioner practicing myoActivation in private, public and primary care. Along with her experience as a palliative care clinician, she cares for populations living with social and health inequities including mental health and addictions. Her research has focused on how myoActivation benefits this population. In 2017 Barb was responsible for introducing myoActivation to the Vancouver Community primary care system. She championed the opening of a pain service in the Downtown Eastside of Vancouver in 2019. Barb has an interest in how historical emotional trauma impacts physical symptoms and uses myoActivation as a tool for addressing this root cause of chronic pain. As a lead instructor for the Anatomic Medicine Foundation, she is keen to teach and mentor other clinicians in learning the myoActivation process.

Dr Gill Lauder MB BCh, FRCA, FRCPC.

Dr Lauder is a pediatric anesthesiologist, complex pediatric pain physician in the Department of Pediatric Anesthesia at BC Children's Hospital (BCCH).

She has worked at BCCH since 2006 in acute, and chronic pediatric pain management. Dr Lauder has 36 years of clinical experience focused to anesthesia and pain management. She has a special interest in pediatric Complex Regional Pain Syndrome (CRPS). She will admit that there have been two "Gamechangers" in her management of chronic pain in youth; one is myoActivation and the other is hypnosis; which TRANCE-forms thoughts, feelings and behaviors. Her current research focuses on demonstrating the benefits of myoActivation; so that more people with lived experience of chronic pain will eventually benefit from this technique.

Fun fact:- She has a shadow but its not black. Her shadow is brown and has four paws; her Pet Therapy dog called Douglas.

Endnotes

[1]   Gillian Lauder, Nicholas West, and Greg Siren, "myoActivation: A Structured Process for Chronic Pain Resolution," in *From Conventional to Innovative Approaches for Pain Treatment*, ed. Marco Cascella, (Intech Open, 2019), http://dx.doi.org/10.5772/intechopen.84377.

[2]   Gillian R. Lauder, Jack Huang, and Nicholas West, "Unrecognized Myofascial Components of Pediatric Complex Pain: myoActivation, a Structured Solution for Assessment and Management," *Current Trends in Internal Medicine* 1, no. 1 (2019): 001–0016.

[3]   myoActivation®, a Structured Assessment and Therapeutic Process for Adolescents With Myofascial Dysfunction and Chronic Low Back Pain: A Case Series. https://www.cureus.com/articles/278504-myoactivation-a-structured-assessment-and-therapeutic-process-for-adolescents-with-myofascial-dysfunction-and-chronic-low-back-pain-a-case-series#!/.

[4]   Tim Bhatnagar, Farah T. Azim, Mona Behrouzian, Karen Davies, Diane Wickenheiser, Gail Jahren, Nicholas West, Lise Leveille, and Gillian R. Lauder, "Assessing Changes in Range of Motion in Adolescent Patients Undergoing myoActivation® for Chronic Pain Related To Myofascial Dysfunction: A Feasibility Study," *Frontiers in Pain Research* 4 (2023):1225088, https://doi.org/10.3389/fpain.2023.1225088.

5   Jacquieline V. Aredo, Katrina J. Heyrana, Barbara I. Karp, Jay P. Shah, and Pamela Stratton, "Relating Chronic Pelvic Pain and Endometriosis to Signs of Sensitization and Myofascial Pain and Dysfunction," *Seminars in Reproductive Medicine* 35, no. 1 (2017): 88–97, https://doi.org/10.1055/s-0036-1597123.

6   Kathleen Meacham, Andrew Shepherd, Durga P. Mohapatra, and Simon Haroutounian, "Neuropathic Pain: Central vs. Peripheral Mechanisms," *Current Pain and Headache Reports* 21, no. 6 (2017): 28, https://doi.org/10.1007/s11916-017-0629-5.

7   Monavar Hadizadeh, Abbas Rahimi, Mohammad Javaherian, Meysam Velayati, and Jan Dommerholt, "The Efficacy of Intramuscular Electrical Stimulation in the Management of Patients with Myofascial Pain Syndrome: A Systematic Review," *Chiropractical & Manual Therapies* 29, no. 1 (2021): 40, https://doi.org/10.1186/s12998-021-00396-z.

8   Jingyi Wen, Xi Chen, Yong Yang, Jianxin Liu, Enyin Li, Jiaoyu Liu, Ziwei Zhou, Weihua Wu, and Kai He, "Acupuncture Medical Therapy and Its Underlying Mechanisms: A Systematic Review," *American Journal of Chinese Medicine* 49, no. 1 (2021): 1–23, https://doi.org/10.1142/s0192415x21500014.

9   Rosa A. Hauser, Johanna B. Lackner, Danielle Steilen-Matias, David K. Harris, "A Systematic Review of Dextrose Prolotherapy for Chronic Musculoskeletal Pain," *Clinical Medicine Insights: Arthritis and Musculoskeletal Disorders* 9 (2016): 139–159, https://doi.org/10.4137/cmamd.s39160.

10   Barbara Cagnie, Vincent Dewitte, Tom Barbe, Frank Timmermans, Nicolas Delrue, and Mira Meeus, "Physiologic Effects of Dry Needling," *Current Pain and Headache Reports* 17, no. 8 (2013): 348, https://doi.org/10.1007/s11916-013-0348-5.

11   Marcos J. Navarro-Santana, Jorge Sanchez-Infante, César Fernández-de-Las-Peñas, Joshua A. Cleland, Patricia Martín-Casas, and Gustavo Plaza-Manzano, "Effectiveness of Dry

Needling for Myofascial Trigger Points Associated with Neck Pain Symptoms: An Updated Systematic Review and Meta-Analysis," *Journal of Clinical Medicine* 9, no. 10 (2020): 3300, https://doi.org/10.3390/jcm9103300.

12   Mehrad Bahramian, Narges Dabbaghipour, Amir Aria, Bahareh Sajadi Moghadam Fard Tehrani, and Jan Dommerholt, "Efficacy of Dry Needling in Treating Scars Following Total Hip Arthroplasty: A Case Report," *Medical Journal of the Islamic Republic of Iran* 20, no. 23 (2022): 156, https://doi.org/10.47176/mjiri.36.156.

13   Robert D. Gerwin, "Diagnosis of Myofascial Pain Syndrome," *Physical Medicine and Rehabilitation Clin of North America* 25, no. 2 (2014): 341–355, https://doi.org/10.1016/j.pmr.2014.01.011.

14   Lynn H. Gerber, Jay Shah, William Rosenberger, Kathryn Armstrong, Diego Turo, Paul Otto, Juliana Heimur, Nikki Thaker, and Siddhartha Sikdar,"Dry Needling Alters Trigger Points in the Upper Trapezius Muscle and Reduces Pain in Subjects with Chronic Myofascial Pain," *Physical Medicine and Rehabilitation* 7, no. 7 (2015): 711–718, https://doi.org/10.1016/j.pmrj.2015.01.020.

15   Jay P. Shah, Nikki Thaker, Juliana Heimur, Jacqueline V. Aredo, Siddhartha Sikdar, and Lynn Gerber, "Myofascial Trigger Points Then and Now: A Historical and Scientific Perspective." *Physical Medicine and Rehabilitation* 7, no. 7 (2015): 746–761, https://doi.org/10.1016/j.pmrj.2015.01.024.

16   Barbara Cagnie, Tom Barbe, Eline De Ridder, Jessica Van Oosterwijck, Ann Cools, and Lieven Danneels, "The Influence of Dry Needling of the Trapezius Muscle on Muscle Blood Flow and Oxygenation," *Journal of Manipulative & Physiological Therapeutics* 35, no. 9 (2012): 685–691, https://doi.org/10.1016/j.jmpt.2012.10.005.

17   Sadia Ahsin, Salman Saleem, Ahsin Mazoor Bhatti, Ray K. Iles, and Mohammad Aslam, "Clinical and Endocrinological

Changes after Electro-acupuncture Treatment in Patients with Osteoarthritis of the Knee," *Pain* 147, no. 1–3 (2009):60–66, https://doi.org/10.1016/j.pain.2009.08.004.

18 Saime Ay, Deniz Evcik, and Birkan Sonel Tur, "Comparison of Injection Methods in Myofascial Pain Syndrome: A Randomized Controlled Trial," *Clinical Rheumatology* 29, no. 1 (2010): 19–23, https://doi.org/10.1007/s10067-009-1307-8.

19 Gyanesh M. Tripathi, Usha K. Misra, Jayantee Kalita, Varun K. Singh, and Abhilasha Tripathi, "Effect of Exercise on β-Endorphin and Its Receptors in Myasthenia Gravis Patients," *Molecular Neurobiology* 60, 6. (2023): 3010–3019, https://doi.org/10.1007/s12035-023-03247-5.

20 Adele Waters, "Depression and the Importance of Hope," *Veterinary Record* 184, no. 15 (2019): 457, https://doi.org/10.1136/vr.l1735.

21 Marco Barbero, Alessandro Schneebeli, Eva Koetsier, and Paolo Maino, "Myofascial Pain Syndrome and Trigger Points: Evaluation and Treatment in Patients with Musculoskeletal Pain," *Current Opinion in Supportive and Palliative Care* 13, no. 3 (2019): 270–276, https://doi.org/10.1097/spc.0000000000000445.

22 Petra Valouchová and Karel Lewit, "Surface Electromyography of Abdominal and Back Muscles in Patients with Active Scars," *Journal of Bodywork and Movement Therapies* 13, no. 3 (2009): 262–267, https://doi.org/10.1016/j.jbmt.2008.04.033; Kay-Hendrik Busch, Antigona Aliu, Nicole Walezko, and Matthias Aust, "Medical Needling: Effect on Skin Erythema of Hypertrophic Burn Scars," *Cureus* 10, no. 9 (2018):e3260, https://doi.org/10.7759/cureus.3260.

23 Yenugandula Vijaya Lakshmi, Lingaladinne Swetha Reddy, Kolli Naga Neelima Devi, Kuchimanchi Phani Kumar, Gandikota Guru Karthik, Pandi Srinivas Chakravarthy, and Kondrakunta Nageswar Rao, "Evaluation of Microneedling Therapy in Management of

Facial Scars," *Journal of Craniofacial Surgery* 31, no. 2 (2020): e214–e217, https://doi.org/10.1097/scs.0000000000006145.

24   R. Brannon Claytor, Casey Gene Sheck, and Vinod Chopra, "Microneedling Outcomes in Early Postsurgical Scars," *Plastic and Reconstructive Surgery* 150, no. 3 (2022): 557e–561e, https://doi.org/10.1097/prs.0000000000009466.

25   Afsaneh Moosaei Saein, Ziaeddin Safavi-Farokhi, Atefeh Aminianfar, and Marzieh Mortezanejad, "The Effect of Dry Needling on Pain, Range of Motion of Ankle Joint, and Ultrasonographic Changes of Plantar Fascia in Patients with Plantar Fasciitis," *Journal of Sport Rehabilitation* 31, no. 3 (2022): 299–304, https://doi.org/10.1123/jsr.2021-0156.

26   Gillian Lauder and Nicholas West, "Clinical Insights into the Importance of Scars and Scar Release in Paediatric Chronic Myofascial Pain," in *Pain Management - Practices, Novel Therapies and Bioactives*, eds. Viduranga Yashasvi Waisundara, Ines Banjari and Jelena Balkić (IntechOpen, 2021), http://dx.doi.org/10.5772/intechopen.93525.

27   Alfonse T. Masi, Sona Kamat, Richard Gajdosik, Naila Ahmad, and Jean C. Aldag, "Muscular Hypertonicity: A Suspected Contributor to Rheumatological Manifestations Observed in Ambulatory Practice," *European Journal of Rheumatology* 2, no. 2 (2015): 66–72, https://doi.org/10.5152/eurjrheum.2015.0119.

28   Kelly A. Pollak, Jeffrey D. Swenson, Timothy A. Vanhaitsma, Ronald W. Hughen, Daehyun Jo, Andrea T. White, Kathleen C. Light, Petra Schweinhardt, Markus Amann, and Alan R. Light, "Exogenously Applied Muscle Metabolites Synergistically Evoke Sensations of Muscle Fatigue and Pain in Human Subjects," *Experimental Physiology* 99, no. 2 (2014): 368–380, https://doi.org/10.1113/expphysiol.2013.075812.

29   Nipaporn Akkarakittichoke, Pooriput Waongenngarm, and Prawit Janwantanakul, "The Effects of Active Break and Postural

Shift Interventions on Recovery from and Recurrence of Neck and Low Back Pain in Office Workers: A 3-Arm Cluster-Randomized Controlled Trial," *Musculoskeletal Science & Practice* 58 (202): 102451, https://doi.org/10.1016/j.msksp.2021.102451.

[30] Erika Zemková and Ludmila Zapletalová, "The Role of Neuromuscular Control of Postural and Core Stability in Functional Movement and Athlete Performance," *Frontiers in Physiology* 13 (2022): 796097, https://doi.org/10.3389/fphys.2022.796097.

[31] Sue Adstrum, Gil Hedley, Robert Schleip, Carla Stecco, and Can A. Yucesoy, "Defining the Fascial System," *Journal of Bodywork and Movement Therapies* 21, no. 1 (2017):173–177, https://doi.org/10.1016/j.jbmt.2016.11.003.

[32] Caterina Fede, Carmelo Pirri, Changlei Fan, Lucia Petrelli, Diego Guidolin, Raffaele De Caro, and Carla Stecco, "A Closer Look at the Cellular and Molecular Components of the Deep/Muscular Fasciae," *International Journal of Molecular Science* 22 (2021): 1411, https://doi.org/10.3390/ijms22031411.

[33] Carla Stecco, Caterina Fede, Veronica Macchi, Andrea Porzionato, Lucia Petrelli, Carlo Biz, Robert Stern, and Raffaele De Caro, "The Fasciacytes: A New Cell Devoted to Fascial Gliding Regulation," *Clinical Anatomy* 31, no. 5 (201): 667–676, https://doi.org/10.1002/ca.23072.

[34] D. McCombe, T. Brown, J. Slavin, and W. A. Morrison, "The Histochemical Structure of the Deep Fascia and Its Structural Response to Surgery," *Journal of Hand Surgery: British Volume* 26, no. 2 (2001): 89–97, https://doi.org/10.1054/jhsb.2000.0546.

[35] Carlos Cruz-Montecinos, Alberto González Blanche, David López Sánchez, Maurico Cerda, Rodolfo Sanzana-Cuche, and Antonio Cuesta-Vargas, "In Vivo Relationship between Pelvis Motion and Deep Fascia Displacement of the Medial Gastrocnemius:

Anatomical and Functional Implications," *Journal of Anatomy* 227, no. 5 (2015): 665–572, https://doi.org/10.1111/joa.12370.

36   Jan Wilke, Robert Schleip, Can A. Yucesoy, and Winfried Banzer, "Not Merely a Protective Packing Organ? A Review of Fascia and Its Force Transmission Capacity," *Journal of Applied Physiology* 124, no. 1 (1985): 234–244, https://doi.org/10.1152/japplphysiol.00565.2017.

37   Bruno Bordoni, Fabiola Marelli, Bruno Morabito, and Beatrice Sacconi, "The Indeterminable Resilience of the Fascial System," *Journal of Integrative Medicine* 15, no. 5 (2017): 337–343, https://doi.org/10.1016/S2095-4964(17)60351-0.

38   Yuya Kodama, Shin Masuda, Toshinori Ohmori, Akhiro Kanamaru, Masato Tanaka, Tomoyoshi Sakaguchi, and Masami Nakagawa, "Response to Mechanical Properties and Physiological Challenges of Fascia: Diagnosis and Rehabilitative Therapeutic Intervention for Myofascial System Disorders," *Bioengineering (Basel)* 10, no. 4 (2023): 474, https://doi.org/10.3390/bioengineering10040474.

39   Mark J. Smeulders, Michiel Kreulen, J. Joris Hage, Peter A. Huijing, and Chantal M. van der Horst, "Spastic Muscle Properties Are Affected by Length Changes of Adjacent Structures," *Muscle & Nerve* 32, no. 2 (2005): 208–215, https://doi.org/10.1002/mus.20360.

40   A. Schilder, U. Hoheisel, W. Magerl, J. Benrath, T. Klein, R.-D. Treede, "Tiefe Gewebe und Rückenschmerzen: Reizung der Fascia thoracolumbalis durch hypertone Kochsalzlösung [Deep Tissue and Back Pain: Stimulation of the Thoracolumbar Fascia with Hypertonic Saline]," *Schmerz* 28, no.1 (2014): 90–92, https://doi.org/10.1007/s00482-013-1373-3.

41   Annemarie Galasso, Ivan Urits, Daniel An, Diep Nguyen, Matthew Borchart, Cyrus Yazdi, Laxmaiah Manchikanti, Rachel J. Kaye, Alan D. Kaye, Ken F. Mancuso, and Omar Viswanath,

"A Comprehensive Review of the Treatment and Management of Myofascial Pain Syndrome," *Current Pain and Headache Reports* 24, no. 8 (2020): 43, https://doi.org/10.1007/s11916-020-00877-5.

42 Derrick G. Sueki, Joshua A. Cleland, and Robert S. Wainner, "A Regional Interdependence Model of Musculoskeletal Dysfunction: Research, Mechanisms, and Clinical Implications," *Journal of Manual & Manipulative Therapy* 21, no. 2 (2013): 90–102, https://doi.org/10.1179/2042618612Y.0000000027.

43 Bruno Bordoni, Kavin Sugumar, and Matthew Varacallo, "Muscle Cramps," *StatPearls* 2023.

44 Sarah Money, "Pathophysiology of Trigger Points in Myofascial Pain Syndrome," *Journal of Pain and Palliative Care Pharmacotherapy* 3, no. 2 (2017): 158–159, https://doi.org/10.1080/15360288.2017.1298688.

45 Bruno Bordoni and Emiliano Zanier, "Skin, Fascias, and Scars: Symptoms and Systemic Connections," *Journal of Multidisciplinary Healthcare* 7 (2013): 11–24, https://doi.org/10.2147/JMDH.S52870.

46 Paolo Tozzi, "Does Fascia Hold Memories?" *Journal of Bodywork and Movement Therapies* 18, no. 2 (2014): 259–265, https://doi.org/10.1016/j.jbmt.2013.11.010.

47 Vidina Suarez-Rodriguez, Caterine Fede, Carmelo Pirri, Lucia Petrelli, Juan Francisco Loro-Ferrer, David Rodriguez-Ruiz, Raffaele De Caro, and Carla Stecco, "Fascial Innervation: A Systematic Review of the Literature," *International Journal of Molecular Science* 23, no. 10 (2022): 5674, https://doi.org/10.3390/ijms23105674.

48 Vidina Suarez-Rodriguez, Caterine Fede, Carmelo Pirri, Lucia Petrelli, Juan Francisco Loro-Ferrer, David Rodriguez-Ruiz, Raffaele De Caro, and Carla Stecco, "Fascial Innervation: A Systematic Review of the Literature," *International Journal*

of Molecular Science 23, no. 10 (2022): 5674, https://doi.org/10.3390/ijms23105674.

49   Jose M. Garcia, George R. Merriam, Atil Y. Kargi, "Growth Hormone in Aging" In *Endotext*, eds. K. R. Feingold, B. Anawalt, M. R. Blackman MR, et al, (MDText.com, Inc.; 2000).

50   Francis Q. S. Dzakpasu, A. Carver, Christian J. Brakenridge, Flavia Cicuttini, Donna M. Urquhart, Neville Owen, David W. Dunstan, "Musculoskeletal Pain and Sedentary Behaviour in Occupational and Non-occupational Settings: A Systematic Review with Meta-analysis," *International Journal of Behavioral Nutrition and Physical Activity* 18, no. 1 (2021): 159, https://doi.org/1.1186/s12966-021-01191-y.

51   Emily Haesler, ed., *Prevention and Treatment of Pressure Ulcers: Clinical Practice Guideline*, National Pressure Ulcer Advisory Panel, European Pressure Ulcer Advisory Panel and Pan Pacific Pressure Injury Alliance (Cambridge Media: 2014), 97.

52   Roger H. Coletti, "The Ischemic Model of Chronic Muscle Spasm and Pain," *European Journal of Translational Myology* 32, no. 1 (2022): 10323, https://doi.org/10.4081/ejtm.2022.10323.

53   Joanna Kamińska, Tomasz Podgórski, Krzysztof Rachwalski, and Maciej Pawlak, "Does the Minerals Content and Osmolarity of the Fluids Taken during Exercise by Female Field Hockey Players Influence on the Indicators of Water-Electrolyte and Acid-Basic Balance?" *Nutrients* 13, no. 2 (2021): 505, https://doi.org/10.3390/nu13020505.

54   Leslie J. Crofford, "Chronic Pain: "Where the Body Meets the Brain," *Transactions of the American Clinical Climatological Association* 126 (2015): 167–183.

55   Stavros A. Kavouras, "Assessing Hydration Status," *Current Opinion in Clinical Nutrition & Metabolic Care* 5, no. 5 (2002): 519–524, https://doi.org/10.1097/00075197-200209000-00010.

56   Wolfgang Marx, Nicola Veronese, Jaimon T. Kelly, Lee Smith, Meghan Hockey, Sam Collins, Gina L. Trakman, Erin Hoare, Scott B. Teasdale, Alexandra Wade, Melissa Lane, Hajara Aslam, Jessica A. Davis, Adrienne O'Neil, Nitin Shivappa, James R. Hebert, Lauren C. Blekkenhorst, Micheal Berk, Toby Segasby, and Felice Jacka, "The Dietary Inflammatory Index and Human Health: An Umbrella Review of Meta-Analyses of Observational Studies" *Advances in Nutrition* 12, no. 5 (2021): 1681–1690, https://doi.org/10.1093/advances/nmab037.

57   Marta Tristan Asensi, Antonia Napoletano, Francesco Sofi, and Monica Dinu, "Low-Grade Inflammation and Ultra-Processed Foods Consumption: A Review," *Nutrients* 15, no. 6 (2023): 1546, https://doi.org/10.3390/nu15061546.

58   Angela M. Quain and Nancy M. Khardori, "Nutrition in Wound Care Management: A Comprehensive Overview," *Wounds* 27, no. 12 (2015): 327–335.

59   Catrin Herpich, Ursula Müller-Werdan, and Kristina Norman, "Role of Plant-Based Diets in Promoting Health and Longevity," *Maturitas* 165 (2022): 47–51, https://doi.org/10.1016/j.maturitas.2022.07.003.

60   Scott Buesing, Miranda Costa, Ja M. Schilling, and Tobias Moeller-Bertram, "Vitamin B12 as a Treatment for Pain," *Pain Physician* 22, no. 1 (2019): E45–E52.

61   Yvoni Kyriakidou, Carly Wood, Chrystalla Ferrier, Alberto Dolci, and Bradley Elliott, "The Effect of Omega-3 Polyunsaturated Fatty Acid Supplementation on Exercise-Induced Muscle Damage," *Journal of International Society of Sports Nutrition* 18, no. 1 (2021): 9, https://doi.org/10.1186/s12970-020-00405-1.

62   A. Capozzi, G. Scambia, S. Migliaccio, and S. Lello, "Role of Vitamin K2 in Bone Metabolism: A Point of View and a Short Reappraisal of the Literature," *Gynecological Endocrinology* 36, no. 4 (2020): 285–288v10.1080/09513590.2019.1689554.

[63] Yanbin Dong, Haidong Zhu, Li Chen, Ying Huang, William Christen, Nancy R. Cook, Trisha Copeland, Samia Mora, Julie E. Buring, I-Min Lee, Karen H. Costenbader, and JoAnn Manson, "Effects of Vitamin D3and Marine Omega-3 Fatty Acids Supplementation on Biomarkers of Systemic Inflammation: 4-Year Findings from the VITAL Randomized Trial," *Nutrients* 14, no. 24 (2022): 5307, https://doi.org/10.3390/nu14245307.

[64] B. T. Flodmark and G. Aase, "Musculoskeletal Symptoms and Type A Behaviour in Blue Collar Workers," *British Journal of Industrial Medicine* 49, no. 10 (1992): 683–687, https://doi.org/10.1136/oem.49.10.683.

[65] W. Michael Hooten, "Chronic Pain and Mental Health Disorders: Shared Neural Mechanisms, Epidemiology, and Treatment," *Mayo Clinic Proceedings* 91, no. 7 (2016): 955–970, https://doi.org/10.1016/j.mayocp.2016.04.029.

[66] Muhammad Hassan Majeed, Ali Ahsan Ali, and Donna M. Sudak, "Mindfulness-Based Interventions for Chronic Pain: Evidence and Applications," *Asian Journal of Psychiatry* 32 (2018): 79–83, https://doi.org/10.1016/j.ajp.2017.11.025.

[67] Pascaline Langlois, Anaick Perrochon, Romain David, Pierre Rainville, Chantal Wood, Audrey Vanhaudenhuyse, Benjamin Pageaux, Amine Ounajim, Martin Lavallière, Ursula Debarnot, Carlos Luque-Moreno, Manuel Roulaud, Martin Simoneau, Lisa Goudman, Maarten Moens, Philippe Rigoard, and Maxime Billot, "Hypnosis to Manage Musculoskeletal and Neuropathic Chronic Pain: A Systematic Review and Meta-analysis," *Neuroscience & Biobehavioral Reviews* 135 (2022): 104591, https://doi.org/10.1016/j.neubiorev.2022.104591.

[68] Valentina Perciavalle, Marta Blandini, Paola Fecarotta, Andrea Buscemi, Donatella Di Corrado, Luana Bertolo, Fulvia Fichera, and Marinella Coco, "The Role of Deep Breathing on Stress,"

114

Neurological Sciences 38, no. 3 (2017): 451–458, https://doi.org/10.1007/s10072-016-2790-8.

69   Semira Manolaki, Ioannis Gkiatas, Spyridon Sioutis, Jimmy Georgoulis, Andreas F. Mavrogenis, George S. Sapkas, Evangelos Alexopoulos, and Christine Darviri, "Relaxation Techniques in Low Back Pain Patients: A Randomized Controlled Trial," *Journal of Long-Term Effects of Medical Implants* 31, no. 2 (2021): 39–44, https://doi.org/10.1615/JLongTermEffMedImplants.2021037026.

70   Sarah Bannon, Jonathan Greenberg, Ryan A. Mace, Joseph J. Locascio, and Ana-Maria Vranceanu, "The Role of Social Isolation in Physical and Emotional Outcomes among Patients with Chronic Pain," *General Hospital Psychiatry* 69 (2021): 50–54, https://doi.org/10.1016/j.genhosppsych.2021.01.009.

71   Joel Vavrina and Josef Vavrina, "Bruxismus: Einteilung, Diagnostik und Behandlung [Bruxism: Classification, Diagnostics and Treatment]," *Praxis* 109, no. 12 (2020): 973–978, https://doi.org/10.1024/1661-8157/a003517.

72   Victoria Parker and Alison J. Douglas, "Stress in Early Pregnancy: Maternal Neuro-endocrine-immune Responses and Effects," *Journal of Reproductive Immunology* 85, no. 1 (2010): 86–92, https://doi.org/10.1016/j.jri.2009.10.011.

73   Roland Staud, "Peripheral Pain Mechanisms in Chronic Widespread Pain," *Best Practice & Research Clinical Rheumatology* 25, no. 2 (2011): 155–164, https://doi.org/10.1016/j.berh.2010.01.010.

74   Anthony F. Domenichiello and Christopher E. Ramsden, "The Silent Epidemic of Chronic Pain in Older Adults," *Progress in Neuropsychopharmacol and Biological Psychiatry* 93 (2019): 284–290, https://doi.org/10.1016/j.pnpbp.2019.04.006.

75   Elizabeth Whitlock, L. Grisell Diaz-Ramirez, M. Maria Glymour, W. John Boscardin, Kenneth E. Covinsky, and Alexander K. Smith, "Association between Persistent Pain and Memory Decline and Dementia in a Longitudinal Cohort of Elders," *JAMA Internal Medicine* 177, no. 8 (2017): 1146–1153, https://doi.org/10.1001/jamainternmed.2017.1622.

76   Andrea L. Chadwick, Nadra E. Lisha, Micah E. Lubensky, Zubin Dastur, Mitchell Lunn, Juno Obedin-Maliver, and Anesa Flentje, "Localized and Widespread Chronic Pain in Sexual and Gender Minority People—An Analysis of The PRIDE Study," *medRxiv* [Preprint] (2023): 2023.11.27.23299101, https://doi.org/10.1101/2023.11.27.23299101.

77   Viviana Guerrieri, Alberto Polizzi, Laura Caliogna, Alice Maria Brancato, Alessandra Bassotti, Camilla Torriani, Eugenio Jannelli, Mario Mosconi, Federico Alberto Grassi, and Gianluigi Pasta, "Pain in Ehlers-Danlos Syndrome: A Non-diagnostic Disabling Symptom?" *Healthcare (Basel)* 11, no. 7 (2023): 936, https://doi.org/10.3390/healthcare11070936.

78   N. Carbonell-Bobadilla, A. A. Rodríguez-Álvarez, G. Rojas-García, J. A. Barragán-Garfias, M . Orrantia-Vertiz, and R. Rodríguez-Romo,"Síndrome de hipermovilidad articular [Joint Hypermobility Syndrome]," *Acta Ortopédica Mexicana* 34, no. 6 (2020): 441–449.

79   Tim Bhatnagar, Farah T. Azim, Mona Behrouzian, Karen Davies, Diane Wickenheiser, Gail Jahren, Nicholas West, Lise Leveille, and Gillian R. Lauder, "Assessing Changes in Range of Motion in Adolescent Patients Undergoing myoActivation® for Chronic Pain Related To Myofascial Dysfunction: A Feasibility Study," *Frontiers in Pain Research* 4 (2023):1225088, https://doi.org/10.3389/fpain.2023.1225088.

80   See myoAforyouth.com, under patient resources, review myoActivation explained.

81 Gillian R. Lauder, Jack Huang, and Nicholas West, "Unrecognized Myofascial Components of Pediatric Complex Pain: myoActivation, a Structured Solution for Assessment and Management," *Current Trends in Internal Medicine* 1, no. 1 (2019): 001–0016.

82 Gillian Lauder and Nicholas West, "Clinical Insights into the Importance of Scars and Scar Release in Paediatric Chronic Myofascial Pain," in *Pain Management - Practices, Novel Therapies and Bioactives*, eds. Viduranga Yashasvi Waisundara, Ines Banjari and Jelena Balkić (IntechOpen, 2021), http://dx.doi.org/10.5772/intechopen.93525.

83 "Home," MyCarePath.ca, https://mycarepath.ca, last accessed 24 October 2024.

84 Tim Bhatnagar, Farah T. Azim, Mona Behrouzian, Karen Davies, Diane Wickenheiser, Gail Jahren, Nicholas West, Lise Leveille, and Gillian R. Lauder, "Assessing Changes in Range of Motion in Adolescent Patients Undergoing myoActivation® for Chronic Pain Related To Myofascial Dysfunction: A Feasibility Study," *Frontiers in Pain Research* 4 (2023):1225088, https://doi.org/10.3389/fpain.2023.1225088.

85 Paolo Tozzi, "Does Fascia Hold Memories?" *Journal of Bodywork and Movement Therapies* 18, no. 2 (2014): 259–265, https://doi.org/10.1016/j.jbmt.2013.11.010.

86 Jenna R. Gale, Jeremy Y. Gedeon, Christopher J. Donnelly, and Michael S. Gold, "Local Translation in Primary Afferents and Its Contribution to Pain," *Pain* 163, no. 12 (2022): 2302–2314, https://doi.org/10.1097/j.pain.0000000000002658.

87 Debbie L. Morton, Javin S. Sandhu, and Anthony K. Jones, "Brain Imaging of Pain: State of the Art," *Journal of Pain Research* 9 (2016): 613–624, https://doi.org/10.2147/JPR.S60433.

88   J. Douglas Bremner, "Neuroimaging in Posttraumatic Stress Disorder and Other Stress-Related Disorders," *Neuroimaging Clinics of North America* 17, no. 4 (2007): 523–538, ix, https://doi.org/10.1016/j.nic.2007.07.003.

89   B. A. van der Kolk, "The Body Keeps the Score: Memory and the Evolving Psychobiology of Posttraumatic Stress," *Harvard Review of Psychiatry* 1, no. 5 (1994): 253–265, https://doi.org/10.3109/10673229409017088. PMID: 9384857.

Printed in Canada